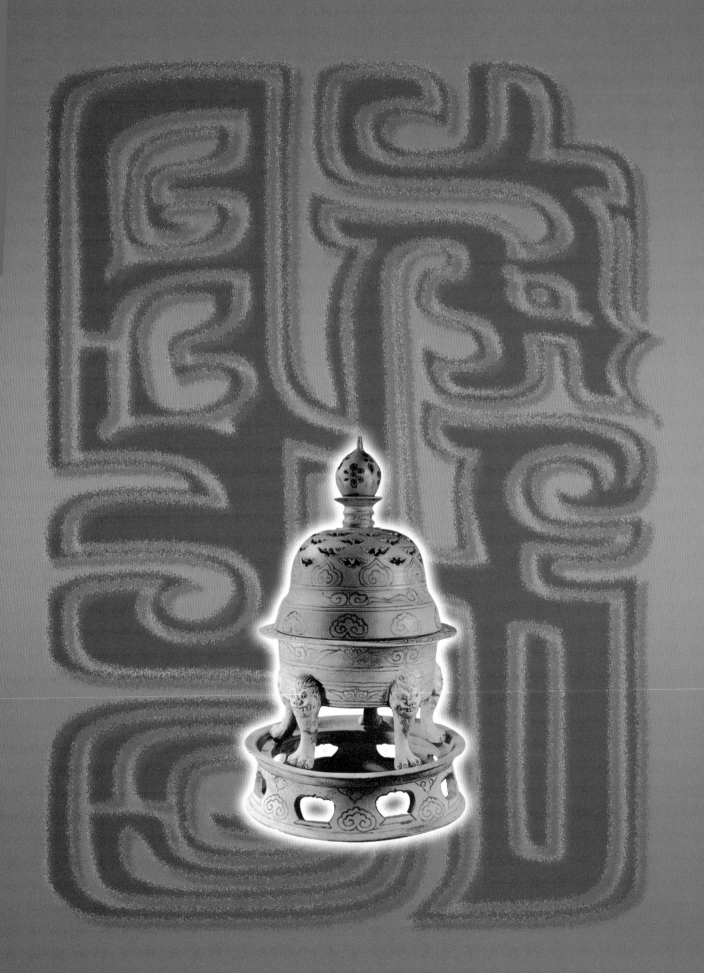

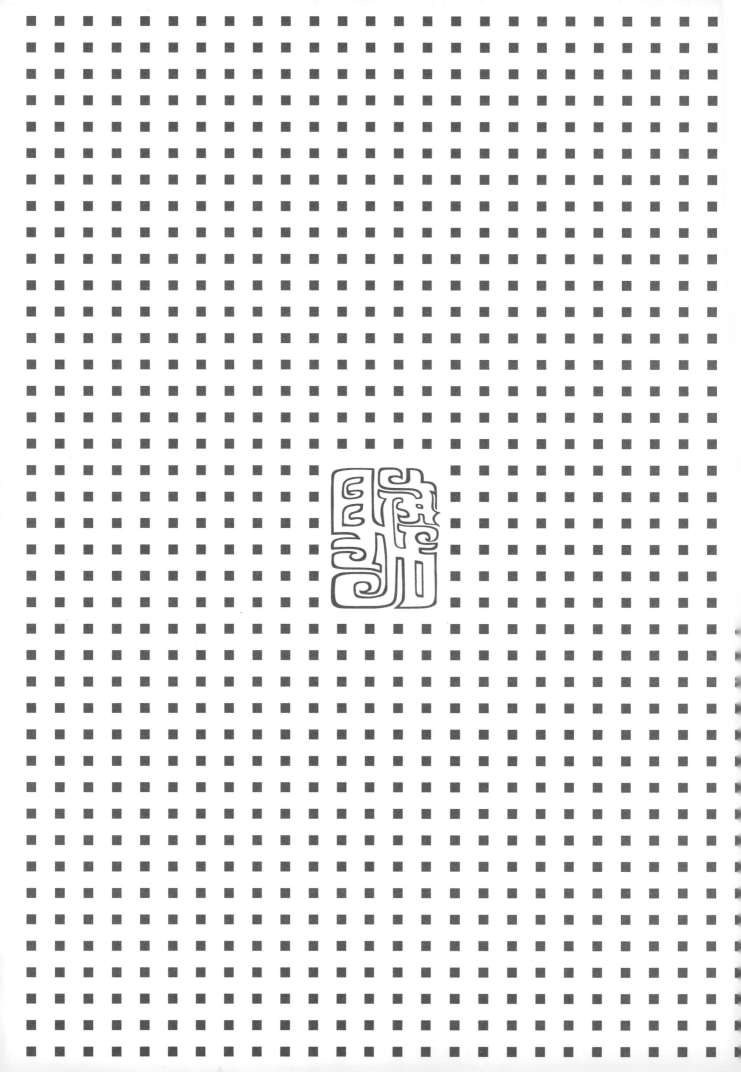

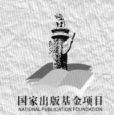

国家出版基金项目
NATIONAL PUBLICATION FOUNDATION

中华医药卫生

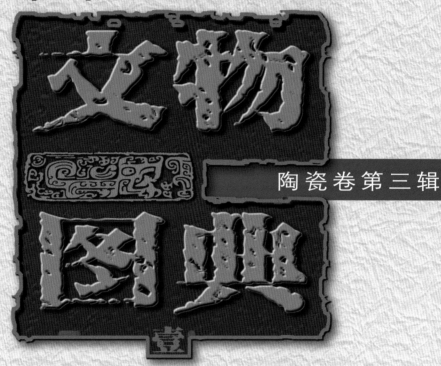

陶瓷卷第三辑

主　编　李经纬　梁　峻　刘学春
总主译　白永权
主　译　陈向京

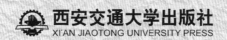

西安交通大学出版社
XI'AN JIAOTONG UNIVERSITY PRESS

图书在版编目 (CIP) 数据

中华医药卫生文物图典 . 1. 陶瓷卷 . 第 3 辑 . / 李经纬，
梁峻，刘学春主编 . — 西安：西安交通大学出版社，2016.12

ISBN 978-7-5605-7030-3

Ⅰ . ①中… Ⅱ . ①李… ②梁… ③刘… Ⅲ . ①中国医药学—
古代陶瓷—中国—图录 Ⅳ . ① R-092 ② K870.2

中国版本图书馆 CIP 数据核字（2015）第 013549 号

书　　名	中华医药卫生文物图典（一）陶瓷卷第三辑
主　　编	李经纬　梁　峻　刘学春
责任编辑	王　磊　李　晶
出版发行	西安交通大学出版社
	（西安市兴庆南路 10 号　邮政编码 710049）
网　　址	http://www.xjtupress.com
电　　话	（029）82668805　82668502（医学分社）
	（029）82668315（总编办）
传　　真	（029）82668280
印　　刷	中煤地西安地图制印有限公司
开　　本	889mm×1194mm　1/16　印张 32.5　字数 491 千字
版次印次	2017 年 12 月第 1 版　2017 年 12 月第 1 次印刷
书　　号	ISBN 978-7-5605-7030-3
定　　价	980.00 元

读者购书、书店添货、如发现印装质量问题，请通过以下方式联系、调换。

订购热线：（029）82665248　（029）82665249

投稿热线：（029）82668805　（029）82668502

读者信箱：medpress@126.com

铭记感受历史

自信自重自强

中华医药卫生文物图典问世书贺

陈可冀 谨题

二〇一九年春月

陈可冀　中国科学院院士、国医大师

精修醫藥衛生文物

圖典功著當代

深究岐黃學術思想

淵源惠澤千秋

中華醫藥衛生文物圖典出版誌慶

丁酉孟秋 孫光榮 敬題於北京

孙光荣 国医大师

中華醫藥衛生文物圖典出版

彰顯中醫藥
文化精神

體現中醫藥
歷史價值

歲次丁酉夏　王琦

王琦　国医大师

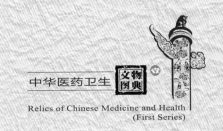

中华医药卫生文物图典（一）
丛书编撰委员会

主　　编　李经纬　梁　峻　刘学春

副主编　廖　果　吴鸿洲　康兴军　和中浚　刘小斌　杨金生

　　　　　郑怀林　徐江雁　白建疆　黄　煌

编　　委　李洪晓　梁永宣　王强虎　董树平　马　健　王　霞

　　　　　张雅宗　朱德明　包哈申　张建青　郑　蓉　庄乾竹

　　　　　李宏红　刘哲峰　王宏才　陈润东

总主译　白永权

主　　译　陈向京　聂文信　范晓晖　温　睿　赵永生　杜彦龙

　　　　　吉　乐　李小棉　郭　梦　陈　曦

副主译（按姓氏音序排列）

　　　　　董艳云　姜雨孜　李建西　刘　慧　马　健　任宝磊

　　　　　任　萌　任　莹　王　颇　习通源　谢皖吉　徐素云

　　　　　许崇钰　许　梅　詹菊红　赵　菲　邹郝晶

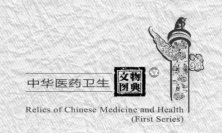

中华医药卫生 文物图典

Relics of Chinese Medicine and Health
(First Series)

本册编撰委员会

主　编　李经纬　梁　峻　刘学春

副主编　廖　果　吴鸿洲　康兴军　和中浚　刘小斌　杨金生

　　　　　郑怀林　徐江雁　白建疆　黄　煌

编　委　李洪晓　梁永宣　王强虎　董树平　马　健　王　霞

　　　　　张雅宗　朱德明　包哈申　张建青　郑　蓉　庄乾竹

　　　　　李宏红　刘哲峰　王宏才　陈润东

总主译　白永权

主　译　陈向京

副主译　许　梅

译　者　邹郝晶　董艳云　郑艳华　许子洋　高　媛　刘妍萌

　　　　　张晓谦　王　丽　王梦杰　王　晨

丛书策划委员会

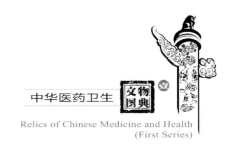

中华医药卫生 文物图典

Relics of Chinese Medicine and Health
(First Series)

序　言

　　探索天、地、人运动变化规律以及"气化物生"过程的相互关系，是人类永恒的课题。宇宙不可逆，地球不可逆，人生不可逆业已成为共识。天地造化形成自然，人类活动构成文化。文物既是文化的载体，又是物化的历史，还是文明的见证。

　　追求健康长寿是人类共同的夙愿。中华民族之所以繁衍昌盛，健康文化起了巨大的推动作用。由于古人谋求生存发展、应对环境变化产生的智慧，大多反映在以医药卫生为核心的健康文化之中，所以，习总书记说："中医药学是中国古代科学的瑰宝，也是打开中华文明宝库的钥匙"。

　　秉持文化大发展、大繁荣理念，中国中医科学院李经纬、梁峻等为负责人的科研团队在完成科技部"国家重点医药卫生文物收集调研和保护"课题获 2005 年度中华中医药学会科技二等奖基础上，又资鉴"夏商周断代工程""中华文明探源工程"等相关考古成果，用有重要价值的新出土文物置换原拍摄质量较差的文物，适当补充民族医药文物，共精选收载 5000 余件。经西安交通大学出版社申报，《中华医药卫生文物图典（一）》（以下简称《图典》）于 2013 年获得了国家出版基金的资助，并经专业翻译团队翻译，使《图典》得以面世。

　　文物承载的信息多元丰富，发掘解读其中蕴藏的智慧并非易事。 医药卫生文物更具有特殊性，除文物的一般属性外，还承载着传统医学发展史迹与促进健康的信息。运用历史唯物主义观察发掘文物信息，善于从生活文物中领悟卫生信息，才能准确解读其功能，也才能诠释其在民生健康中的历史作用，收到以古鉴今之效果。"历史是现实的根源"，任何一个民族都不能割断历史，史料都包含在文化中。"文化是民族的血脉，是人民的精神家园"，文化繁荣才能实现中华民族的伟大复兴。值本《图典》付梓之际，用"梳理文化之脉，必获健康之果"作为序言并和作者、读者共勉！

中央文史研究馆馆员

中国工程院院士　　王永炎

丁酉年仲夏

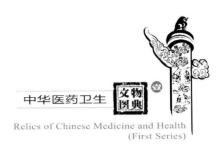

中华医药卫生 文物图典

Relics of Chinese Medicine and Health
(First Series)

前　言

　　文化是相对自然的概念，是考古界常用词汇。文物是文化的重要组成部分，既是文明的物证，又是物化的历史。狭义医药卫生文物是疾病防治模式语境下的解读，而广义医药卫生文物则是躯体、心态、环境适应三维健康模式下的诠释。中华民族是56个民族组成的多元一体大家庭，中华医药卫生文物当然包括各民族的健康文化遗存。

　　天地造化如造山、板块漂移、气候变迁、生物起源进化等形成自然。气化物生莫贵于人，即整个生物进化的最高成果是人类自身。广义而言，人类生存思维留下的痕迹即物质财富和精神财富总和构成文化，其一般的物化形式是视觉感知的文物、文献、胜迹等。其中质变标志明晰的文化如文字、文物、城市、礼仪等可称作文明。从唯物史观视角观察，狭义文化即精神财富，尤其体现人类精、气、神状态的事项，其本质也具有特殊物质属性，如量子也具有波粒二相性，这种粒子也是物质，无非运动方式特殊而已。现代所谓可重复验证的"科学"，事实上也是从文化中分离出来的事项，因此也是一种特殊文化形式。追求健康长寿是人类共同的夙愿。中华民族之所以繁衍昌盛，是因为健康文化异彩纷呈。中华优秀传统医药文化之所以博大精深，是因为其原创思维博大、格物致知精深，所以，习总书记说："中医药学是中国古代科学的瑰宝，也是打开中华文明宝库的钥匙"。

文化既反映时代、地域、民族分布、生产资料来源、技术水平等信息，又反映人类认知水平和生存智慧。发掘解读文物、文献中蕴藏的健康知识和灵动智慧，首先是从事健康工作者的责任和义务。《易经》设有"观"卦，人类作为观察者，不仅要积极收藏展陈文物，而且要善于捕捉文物倾诉的信息，汲取养分，启迪思维，收到古为今用之效果。墨子三表法，首先一表即"本之于古者圣王之事"，也是强调古代史实的重要性。"历史是现实的根源"，现实是未来的基础。任何一个国家、地区、民族都不能割断历史、忽略基础，这个基础就是文化。"文化是民族的血脉，是人民的精神家园"。文化繁荣才能驱动各项事业发展，才能实现中华民族的伟大复兴。

人类从类人猿分化出来。"禄丰古猿禄丰种"是云南禄丰发现的类人猿化石，距今七八百万年。距今 200 万年前人类进入旧石器时代，直立行走，打制石器产生工具意识，管理火种，是所谓"燧人氏"时代。中国留存有更新世早、中期的元谋、蓝田、北京人等遗址。距今 10 万—5 万年前，人类进入旧石器时代中期，即早期智人阶段，脑容量增加，和欧洲、非洲人种相比，原始蒙古人种颧骨前突等，是所谓"伏羲氏"时代。中国发现的马坝、长阳、丁村人等较典型。距今 5 万—1 万年前，人类进入旧石器时代晚期，即晚期智人阶段，细石器、骨角器等遍布全国，山顶洞、柳江、资阳人等较典型。

中石器时代距今约 1 万年，是旧石器时代向新石器时代的短暂过渡期，弓箭发明，狗被驯化。河南灵井、陕西沙苑遗址等作为代表。距今 1 万—公元前 2600 年前后，人类进入新石器时代，磨光石器、烧制陶器，出现农业村落并饲养家畜，是所谓"神农氏"时代。公元前 7000 年以来，在甲、骨、陶、石等载体上出现契刻符号、七音阶骨笛乐器等，反映出人文气息趋浓。公元前 6000—公元前 3500 年的老官台、裴李岗、河姆渡、马家浜、仰韶等文化遗址，彰显出先民围绕生存健康问题所做的各种努力。

公元前 4800 年以来，以关中、晋南、豫西为中心形成的仰韶文化，是中原史前文化的重要标志。以半坡、庙底沟类型为典型，自公元前 3500 年走向繁荣，属于锄耕粟黍稻兼营渔猎饲养猪鸡经济方式，彩陶尤其发达。公元前 4400—公元前 3300 年，长江中游的大溪文化，薄胎彩陶和白陶发达。公元前 4300—公元前 2500 年山东丰岛的大汶口文化，红陶为主。公元前 3500 年前后，辽东的红山文化原始宗教发展。公元前 3300 年以来，长江下游由河姆渡、马家浜文化衍续的良渚文化和陇西的马家窑文化、江淮间的薛家岗文化时趋发达。

公元前 2600—公元前 2000 年，黄河中下游龙山文化群形成，冶铸铜器，制作玉器，土坯、石灰、夯筑技术开始应用。公元前 2697 年，轩辕战败炎帝（有说其后裔）、蚩尤而为黄帝纪元元年。黄帝西巡访贤，"至岐见岐伯，引载而归，访于治道"。其引归地"溱洧襟带于前，梅泰环拱于后"，即今河南新密市古城寨。岐黄答问，构建《黄帝内经》健康知识体系，中华文明从关注民生健康起步。颛顼改革宗教，神职人员出现；帝喾修身节用，帝尧和合百国，舜同律度量衡，大禹疏导治水，中华民族不断繁衍昌盛。

公元前 2070 年，禹之子启以豫西晋南为中心建立夏王朝，二里头青铜文化为其特征，半地穴、窑洞、地面建筑并存。饮食卫生器具、酒器增多。朱砂安神作用在宫殿应用。公元前 1600 年，商灭夏。偃师商城设有铸铜作坊。公元前 1300 年，盘庚迁殷，使用甲骨文。武丁时期青铜浑铸、分铸并存。公元前 1056 年，相传周"文王被殷纣拘于姜里，演《周易》，成六十四卦"。公元前 1046 年，武王克商建周，定都镐京。青铜器始铸长篇铭文，周原发掘出微型甲骨文字。公元前 770 年，平王东迁。虢国铸铜柄铁剑。公元前 753 年，秦国设置史官。公元前 707 年出现蝗灾、公元前 613 年出现"哈雷彗星"，均被孔子载入《春秋》。公元前 221 年，秦始皇统一中国，多元一体民族大家庭形成，中华医药卫生文物异彩纷呈。

中国是治史大国，历来重视发展文化博物事业，1955 年成立卫生部中医研究院时就设置医史研究室，1982 年中国医史文献研究所成立时复建中国医史博物馆研究收藏展陈文物。2000—2003 年，经王永炎院士、姚乃礼院长等呼吁，科技部批准立项，由李经纬、梁峻为负责人的团队完成"国家重点医药卫生文物收集调研和保护"项目任务，受到科技部项目验收组专家的高度评价，获中华中医药学会科技进步二等奖。2013 年，在国家出版基金资助下，课题组对部分文物重新拍摄或必要置换、充实民族医药文物后，由西安交通大学出版社编辑、组聘国内一流翻译团队英译说明文字付梓，受到国家中医药博物馆筹备工作领导小组和办公室的高度重视。

"物以类聚"，《图典》主要依据文物质地、种类分为 9 卷，计有陶瓷，金属，纸质，竹木，玉石、织品及标本，壁画石刻及遗址，少数民族文物，其他，备考等卷。同卷下主要根据历史年代或小类分册设章。每卷下的历史时段不求统一。遵循上述规则将《图典》划分为 21 册，总计收载文物 5000 余件。对每件文物的描述，除质地、规格、馆藏等基本要素外，重点描述其在民生健康中的作用。对少数暂不明确的事项在括号中注明待考。对引自各博物馆的材料除在文物后列出馆藏外，还在书后再次统一列出馆名或参考书目，以充分尊重其馆藏权，也同时维护本典作者的引用权。

21 世纪，围绕人类健康的生命科学将飞速发展，但科学离不开文化，文化离不开文物。发掘文物承载的信息为现实服务，谨引用横渠先生四言之两语："为天地立心，为生民立命"，既作为编撰本《图典》之宗旨，也是我们践行国家"一带一路"倡议的具体努力。希冀通过本《图典》的出版发行，教育国人，提振中华民族精神；走向世界，为人类健康事业贡献力量。

李经纬　梁峻　刘学春

2017 年 6 月于北京

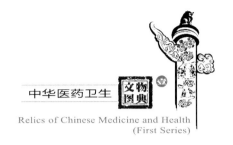

中华医药卫生
Relics of Chinese Medicine and Health
(First Series)

目 录

第二章 隋 唐

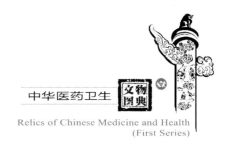

中华医药卫生 文物图典

Relics of Chinese Medicine and Health
(First Series)

Contents

Chapter Two Sui and Tang Dynasty

◆ 第一章　魏晋南北朝

Chapter One　　Wei, Jin and Southern
and Northern Dynasties

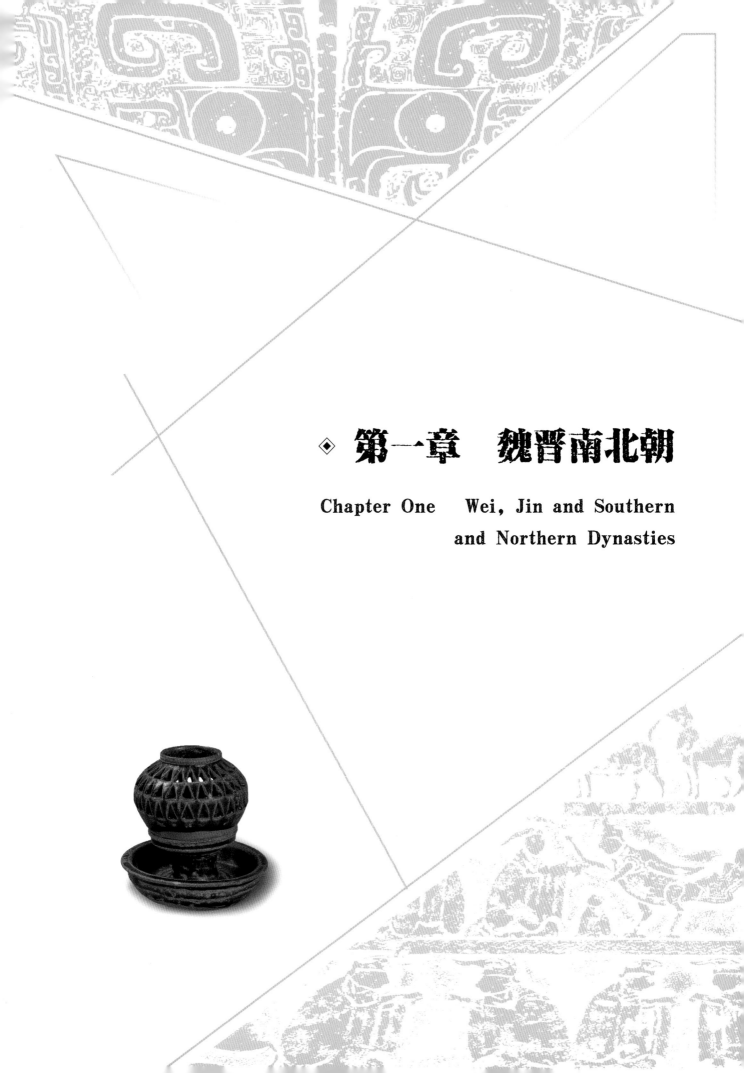

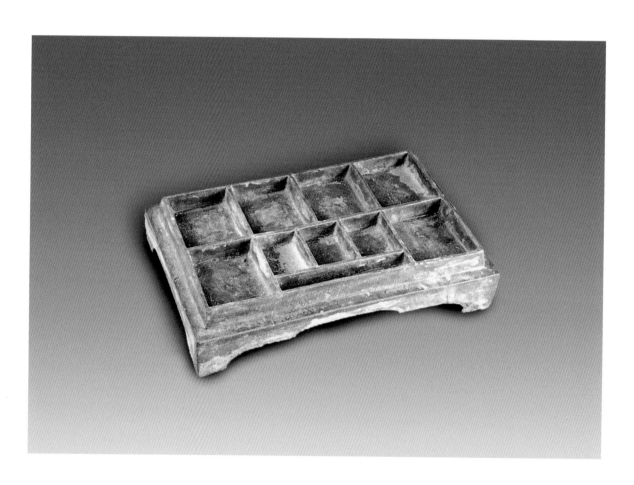

红陶多子盒

三国·魏（220—265）

陶质

长 27.8 厘米，宽 17.8 厘米，高 6.2 厘米

Red Pottery Box with Several Lattices

Three Kingdoms, the State of Wei (220–265)

Pottery

Length 27.8 cm/ Width 17.8 cm/ Height 6.2 cm

泥质红陶胎，器表施以酱红色釉。釉面均匀而稍有光泽。用以盛装果品和点心。器身呈长方形，分成大小不等的 10 个方形小格，所分成的小格可以将食品按质地和类别分置，装满后上部可以加盖扣合。北京市海淀区八里庄曹魏墓出土。

北京大学赛克勒考古与艺术博物馆藏

The box is made of clay with a red pottery body, the surface of which is evenly glazed carmine red with luster. Used for containing fruits and snacks, this rectangle-shaped box is divided into ten little square lattices of varied sizes, in which food of different ingredients and categories could be stored. The lid of the box is used to fasten the box down when it is full. It was excavated from Caowei Mausoleum, Bali Village, Haidian District, Beijing.

Preserved in Arthur M.Sackler Museum of Art and Archaeology at Peking University

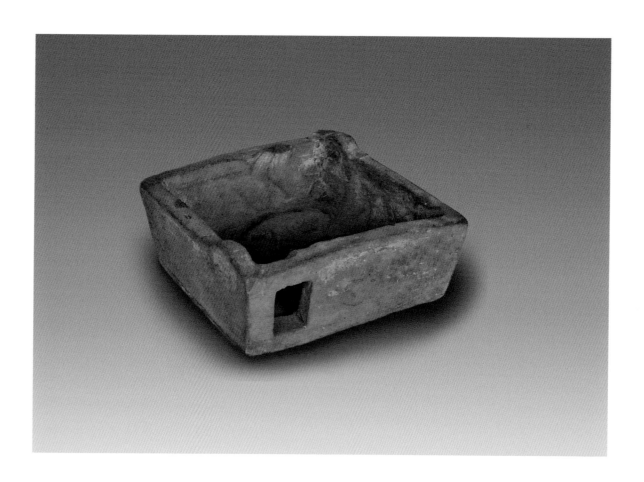

陶猪圈

魏

陶质

边长 14.2 厘米，通高 5.75 厘米

Pottery Pigsty

Wei Dynasty

Pottery

Side Length 14.2 cm/ Height 5.75 cm

该藏灰黑陶制成，猪圈内塑一陶猪。一角有圈门，外部平整，内部粗糙，上口凸凹不平。方形，为丧葬明器。1960 年入藏。保存基本完好。

中华医学会 / 上海中医药大学医史博物馆藏

This pigsty is made from grey-black pottery. A pottery swine is found inside the pigsty and a pen door in the corner. The exterior of the pigsty is smooth while the interior is rough. The square pigsty with an uneven upper surface is a burial object. Collected in the year 1960, this article has been kept intact.

Preserved in Chinese Medical Association/Museum of Chinese Medicine, Shanghai University of Traditional Chinese Medicine

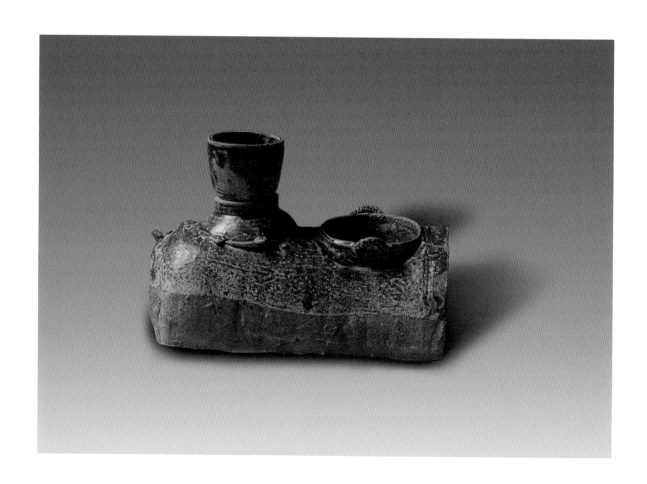

酱褐斑青瓷灶

六朝早期

瓷质

长 26 厘米，通高 16 厘米

Celadon Stove with Caramel-brown Speckles

Early Six Dynasties

Porcelain

Length 26 cm/ Height 16 cm

灰白色胎，酱褐色釉中有黄釉斑，釉层较均匀，略见垂流不及底。器物下部露有紫色粗砂坯胎。灶身呈券顶形，前部开券顶式长方形灶门，尾部有一小孔作烟囱状，灶顶安置一锅，锅有两耳，后灶有一甑，置放于釜上。整体器形为伏虎状。该灶器形规整，做工讲究，不仅能够节约燃料，而且符合热空气流动原理。1996年江宁县江宁镇梅府出土。

江宁博物馆藏

The body of the stove is in the colour of hoary. Yellow speckles scatter on the uniform caramel-brown glaze, which runs downward close to the bottom. Purple grit body is exposed at the lower part of the object. In front of the vaulting-shaped stove body is a rectangular arch door, and a small hole at the tail seems to be the chimney. A double-eared pot is placed on the top of the stove, and a steamer on the cauldron at the back stove. The entire set is in the shape of a squatting tiger. With neat structure and exquisite workmanship, the stove not only saves fuel but also conforms to the principle of hot air-flow. It was unearthed from Meifu Village at Jiangning Town in Jiangning County, Jiangsu Province, in the year 1996.

Preserved in Jiangning Museum

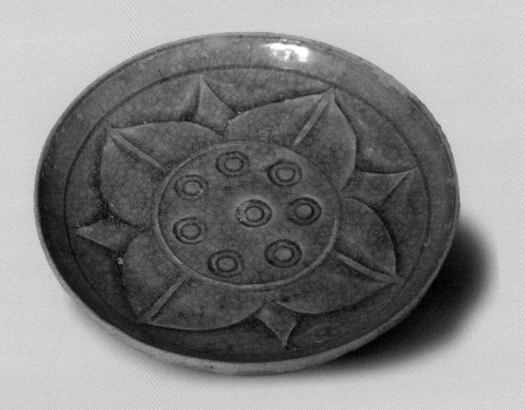

青釉刻花盘

六朝

瓷质

口径 14.2 厘米，高 25 厘米

敛口，浅腹，平底。盘中央刻莲瓣纹，叶肥宽广，盘心加圆圈纹，刻画粗犷有力。全器满釉，仅底足无釉。施釉不匀，釉质润泽，厚处闪青，薄处闪黄，开冰裂纹片。

曾广亿藏

Celadon Plate with Incised Floral Design

Six Dynasties

Porcelain

Mouth Diameter 14.2 cm/ Height 25 cm

This plate is characterized by a contracted mouth, a shallow belly and a flat foot. In the centre of the plate is incised a lotus petal motif with fleshy and broad foliage, and the heart of the plate is decorated with circular patterns. With bold and unrestrained carving and incised motifs, the plate is fully glazed except for the foot. The uneven glaze is smooth and lustrous with ice crack glaze, glittering green in the thick part and yellow in the thin part.

Collected by Zeng Guangyi

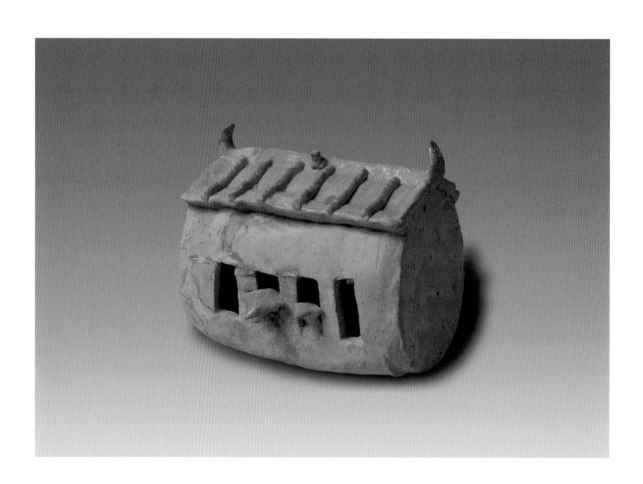

青瓷羊圈

六朝

青瓷质

长 26 厘米，高 18 厘米

Celadon Sheepfold

Six Dynasties

Celadon Porcelain

Length 26 cm/ Height 18 cm

作屋形，正面作栏杆状，羊头从圈内伸出。顶部作两坡顶有瓦垅状饰，脊两端置鸱尾。局部脱釉。丧葬明器。该器有助于人们认识六朝时代南京地区的建筑风格和家畜饲养状况。南京出土。

南京博物院藏

This sheepfold with some glaze scales is in the shape of a house. A row of balusters serves as an open parapet for sheep to crane their necks. The sheepfold has an even-span roof with the corrugated decoration and owl-shaped ridge end. It was utilized as a burial object. This celadon sheepfold gives a clear picture both of the architectural style in Nanjing Area in the Six Dynasties and of cattle breeding at that time. It was excavated from Nanjing, Jiangsu Province. Preserved in Nanjing Museum

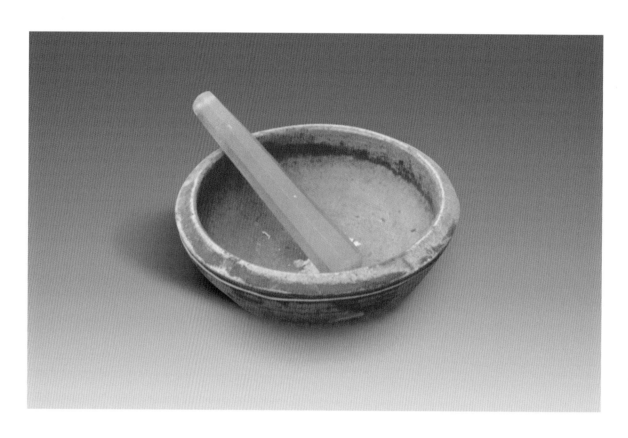

瓷研钵

晋

陶瓷质

口外径 11.4 厘米，底径 7.6 厘米，腹径 13.1 厘米，
通高 4.1 厘米，腹深 3.4 厘米，重 308 克
瓷研钵带杵，瓷质钵，玉杵，用于研细药物。

广东中医药博物馆藏

Porcelain Mortar

Jin Dynasty

Porcelain

Mouth Outer Diameter 11.4 cm/ Bottom Diameter
7.6 cm/ Belly Diameter 13.1 cm/ Height 4.1 cm/
Depth 3.4 cm/ Weight 308 g

The whole set contains a porcelain mortar and a
jade pestle used to crush or grind drug ingredients.

Preserved in Guangdong Chinese Medicine Museum

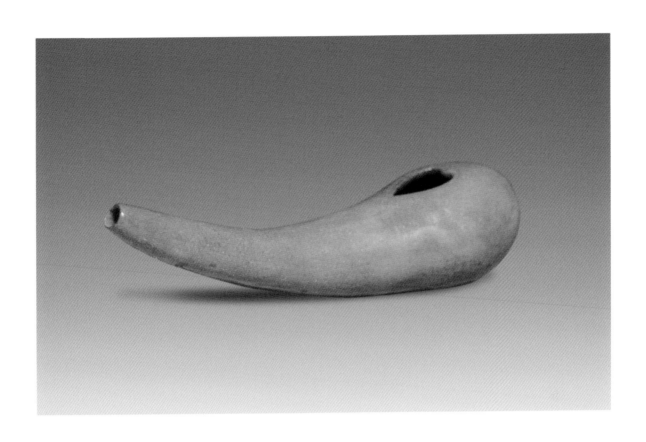

灌药器

晋

瓷质

长 25 厘米，口径 1 厘米，腹径 7.2 厘米

用于灌装备用药水，一般用于外科、眼科。侯宝璋捐献。

首都博物馆藏

Drencher

Jin Dynasty

Porcelain

Length 25 cm/ Mouth Diameter 1 cm/ Belly Diameter 7.2 cm

The drencher was utilized for storing alternate medicine potion, commonly used in surgery and ophthalmology. This object is donated by Hou Baozhang.

Preserved in the Capital Museum

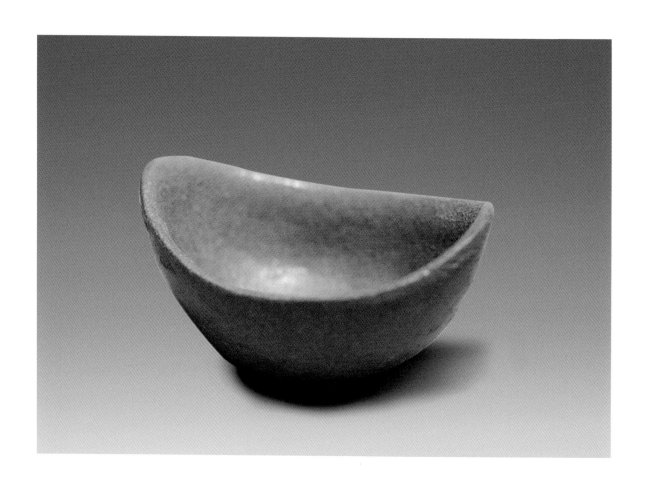

洗眼杯

晋

瓷质

长 5.5 厘米，宽 4 厘米，高 3 厘米

Eye-washing Cup

Jin dynasty

Porcelain

Length 5.5 cm/ Width 4 cm/ Height 3 cm

杯口上沿弧形，恰与人眼眶相吻合。用于外治眼疾。侯宝璋捐献。

首都博物馆藏

The arc-shaped edge of the cup mouth fits human orbit exactly. The cup was used for the treatment of eye diseases. It was donated by Hou Baozhang.

Preserved in the Capital Museum

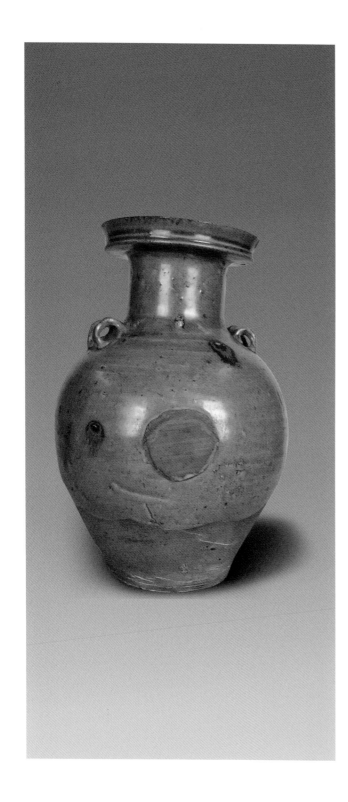

四耳瓷药壶

晋

瓷质

口内径 7.7 厘米，口外径 13.9 厘米， 腹围
67 厘米，通高 29 厘米

Drug Pot with Four Ears

Jin Dynasty

Porcelain

Inner Mouth Diameter 7.7 cm/ Outer Mouth
Diameter 13.9 cm/ Belly Diameter 67 cm/
Height 29 cm

该藏罐腹以上施草绿釉，下部及底无釉，肩部置四系，罐腹处还有胎补一处，平底无款，无盖。壶形，为煎药器具。1958 年入藏。保存基本完好，口残。

中华医学会 / 上海中医药大学医史博物馆藏

The upper abdomen of the pot is glazed prasinous, while the underpart and the bottom are unglazed. On the shoulder can be found four rings, and on the belly a mark of restoration. No inscription is found on the flat bottom, nor any cover on the top. It was collected in the year 1958 and kept in good condition. The pot, with its mouth damaged, was an implement for decocting medicinal herbs.

Preserved in Chinese Medical Association/ Museum of Chinese Medicine, Shanghai University of Traditional Chinese Medicine

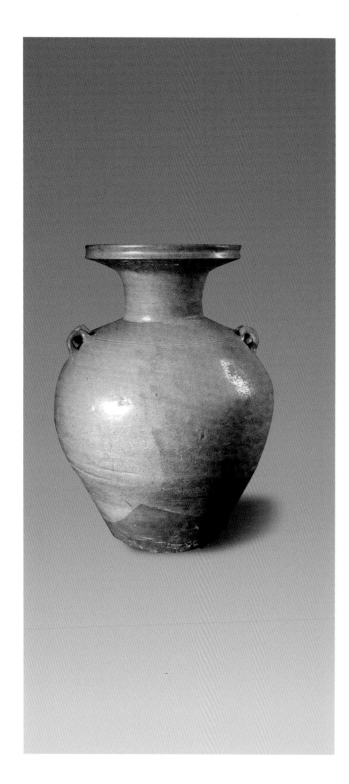

四耳壶

晋

瓷质

口径 16 厘米，底径 12 厘米，高 30.5 厘米

Pot with Four Ears

Jin Dynasty

Porcelain

Mouth Diameter 16 cm/ Bottom Diameter 12 cm/

Height 30.5 cm

据《支那青瓷史稿》载，日本法隆寺发现的越窑药壶同此，故此壶当也用于盛放药物。浙江绍兴九岩镇出土。

上海中医药博物馆藏

This pot shares common features with the drug pots unearthed from Hōryū-ji, a Buddhist temple in Japan, according to *The History of Chinese Celadon*. They were made in Yue kiln. This pot is believed to be utilized for storing drugs. It was excavated from Jiuyan Town of Shaoshing, Zhejiang Province.
Preserved in Shanghai Museum of Traditional Chinese Medicine

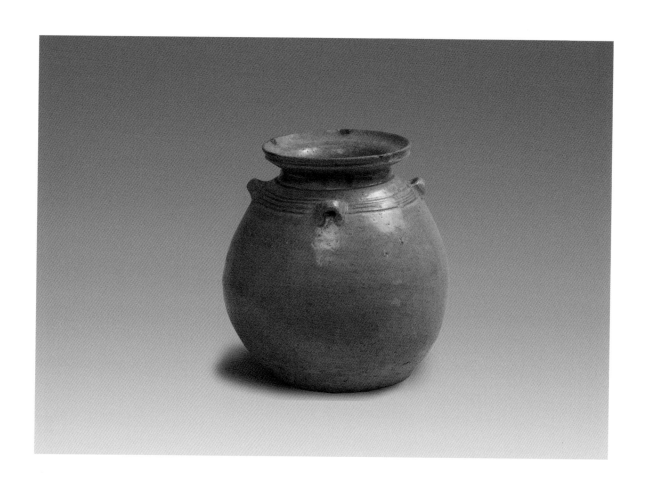

垂腹盘口壶

东晋

瓷质

Plate-shaped Pot with Vertical Abdomen

Eastern Jin Dynasty

Porcelain

浅盘口，短直颈，溜肩，垂腹，平底微内凹，肩部饰凹弦纹四道，其上压塑横系，泥条盘筑，两两相对，通体罩青绿釉，微闪黄，胎釉结合牢固，口沿点缀酱釉褐斑。

南京王谢古陈列馆藏

The pot is designed with a shallow dish-shaped mouth, a short and straight neck, a sloping shoulder, a vertical abdomen and a slightly concaved bottom. The shoulder is decorated with four bands of string patterns, on which four symmetrical rings formed by clay-strip are compressed and moulded. The entire pot is coated with bluish green glaze, with a slightly yellowish shine. The body and the glaze are in firm combination, with brown-glazed speckles embellished at the rim.

Preserved in Exhibition Hall of Former Residence of Wangxie in Nanjing

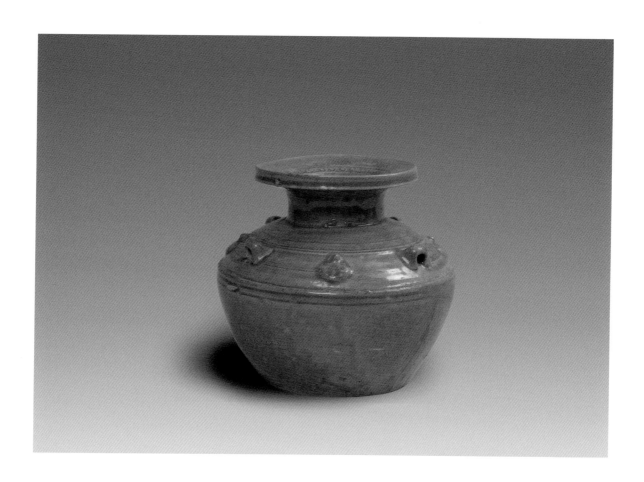

青釉佛饰瓷口壶

西晋

瓷质

口径 11 厘米，腹径 17 厘米，底径 10.5 厘米，高 14.3 厘米

Celadon Pot with Buddhist Symbols

Western Jin Dynasty

Porcelain

Mouth Diameter 11 cm/ Belly Diameter 17 cm/ Bottom Diameter 10.5 cm/ Height 14.3 cm

浅盘口，直筒式颈，斜折肩，平底。通体施草釉，肩部饰弦纹七道，在第三与第五道弦纹之间有四只泥条半环横系。四系间贴塑佛像四个，佛像均结跏趺坐于莲花座上。

南京王谢古居陈列馆藏

The shallow plate-mouthed pot has a straight neck, an obliquely angular shoulder and a flat bottom. The entire pot is coated with grass green glaze. The shoulder is decorated with seven bands of string patterns, and four semi-circular clay-strip rings are placed horizontally between the third and the fifth string. Sitting on the lotus pedestal with crossed legs, four Buddha statues are pasted on the shoulder of the pot, spaced apart by the four rings.

Preserved in Exhibition Hall of Former Residence of Wangxie in Nanjing

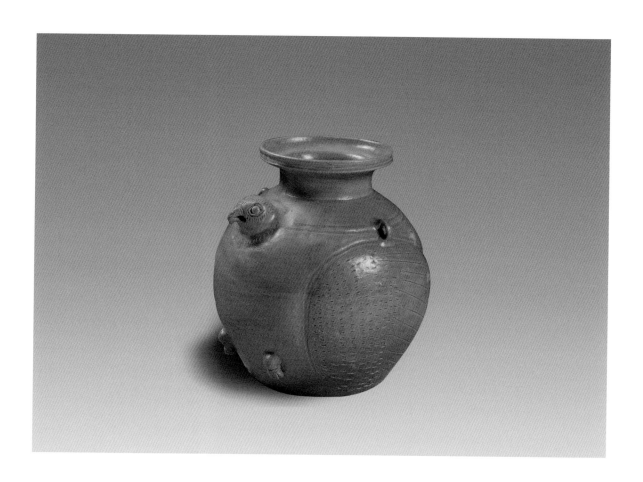

青釉鹰形瓷盘口壶

西晋

瓷质

口径 10.9 厘米，高 11.9 厘米

Eagle-shaped Celadon Pot with Plate-shaped Mouth

Western Jin Dynasty

Porcelain

Mouth Diameter 10.9 cm/ Height 11.9 cm

浅灰色胎，青灰釉。浅盘口，短颈，鼓腹，平底。肩堆塑鹰首，圆目勾喙。腹两侧刻画双翼，胫贴附双足及鹰尾。该器将鹰的器官巧妙地置于盘口壶上，仿佛一只栖于枝头的鹰，双目圆睁，眈眈待食。用鹰装饰盘口壶在目前考古中仅见，装饰设计清新，实用与美观并重，弥足珍贵。南京板桥石闸湖汝阴太守墓出土。

南京博物院藏

This pot has a pale body, a shallow plate-shaped mouth, a short neck, a drum abdomen and a flat bottom. An eagle head, with round eyes and hooked beak, is moulded on the shoulder of the pot. The eagle's wings are incised on the abdomen, with its feet and a tail attached to the lower part of the pot. The body of the round-eyed eagle are tactfully placed onto the pot, like one perching on branches, ready for a hunt. This is a unique plate-shaped mouth pot in the form of an eagle. Novelly designed, this pot is of both pragmatic and aesthetic values. It was unearthed from the tomb of Prefecture Ruyin at Stone Gate Lake in Banqiao Road in Nanjing.
Preserved in Nanjing Museum

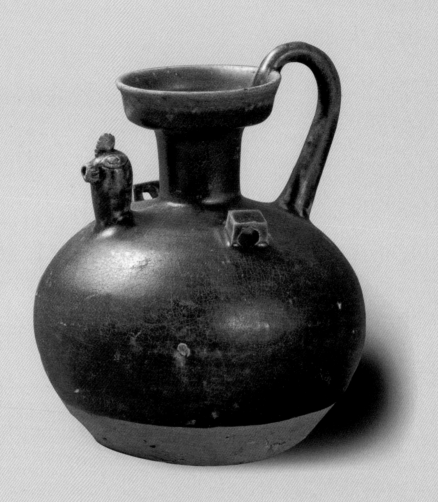

褐釉瓷鸡首壶

东晋

瓷质

口径 7 厘米，底径 9 厘米，高 14.8 厘米

Brown-glazed Ewer with Chicken-head Spout

Eastern Jin Dynasty

Porcelain

Mouth Diameter 7 cm/ Bottom Diameter 9 cm/ Height 14.8 cm

盘口，直颈，鼓腹，平底略内凹，壶嘴作鸡首状，塑鸡冠、眼、口和颈，壶嘴与腹相通，另一侧有圆弧形柄，上接口，下连肩。壶两边附桥形系。此壶施酱釉，釉色浑厚匀净，是一件十分珍贵的德清窑瓷器的精品。南京江宁县下坊村出土。

南京博物院藏

The ewer has a plate-shaped mouth, a straight neck, a globular body and a bottom slightly concaved inward. The spout is made in the shape of a chicken's head, with moulded beak, comb, eyes, and neck. The spout interconnects with the abdomen. On the other side is of the ewer placed a curved handle connected upward to the mouth and downward to the shoulder. Bridge-shaped ears are attached to both sides of the ewer. This object, uniformly and neatly glazed with thick brown, is an exquisite piece of work made in Deqing kiln. It was unearthed from Xiafang Village at Jiangning County in Nanjing.

Preserved in Nanjing Museum

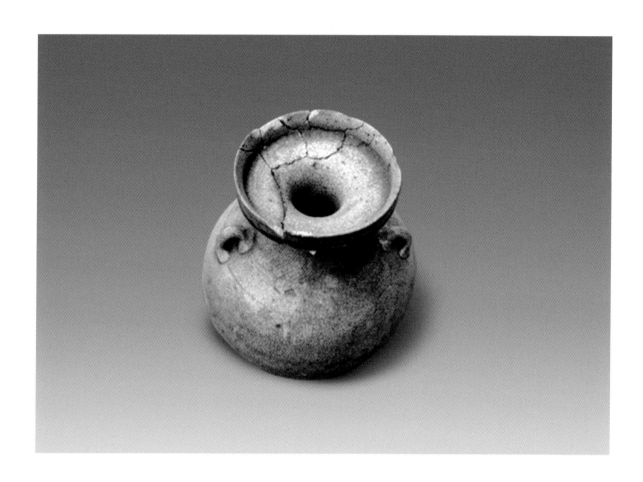

青瓷双系瓷壶

晋

瓷质

上口径 11.8 厘米，壶身径 17.2 厘米，底径 11.3 厘米，高 20.2 厘米，壶深 18.5 厘米

Celadon Pot with Two Rings

Jin Dynasty

Porcelain

Mouth Diameter 11.8 cm/ Belly Diameter 17.2 cm/ Bottom Diameter 11.3 cm/ Height 20.2 cm/ Depth 18.5 cm

肩有系，鼓腹，颈细，盘口。储容器。

广东中医药博物馆藏

With handles on the shoulder, the pot is designed with a drum abdomen, a thin neck and a plate-shaped mouth. It served as a container.

Preserved in Guangdong Chinese Medicine Museum

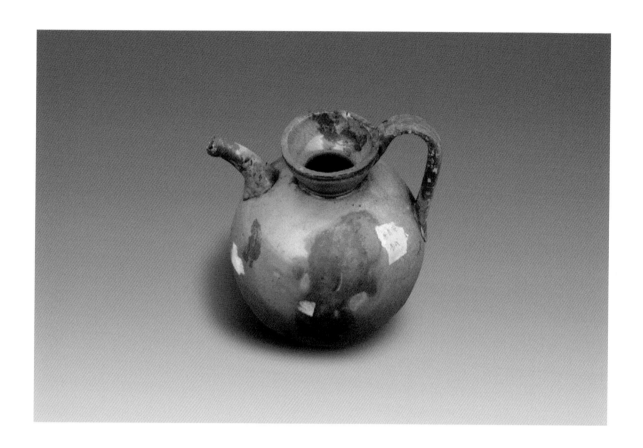

青瓷壶

晋

瓷质

外口径 6.6 厘米，腹径 13.05 厘米，底径 6.6 厘米，通高 16.1 厘米，腹深 15.5 厘米，重 810 克

Celadon Ewer

Jin Dynasty

Porcelain

Outer Diameter 6.6 cm/ Belly Diameter 13.05 cm/ Bottom Diameter 6.6 cm/ Height 16.1 cm/ Depth 15.5 cm/
Weight 810 g

带把，壶嘴，平底。生活用品。

广东中医药博物馆藏

This porcelain ewer, with a handle, a spout and a flat bottom, was a household utensil.

Preserved in Guangdong Chinese Medicine Museum

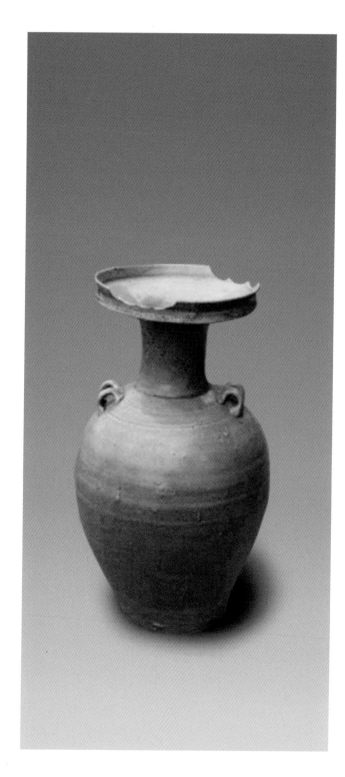

青瓷四系壶

晋

瓷质

口外径 15 厘米，底径 10.9 厘米，通高 33.3 厘米，腹深 19.5 厘米，重 2600 克

Celadon Pot with Four Rings

Jin Dynasty

Porcelain

Outer Diameter 15 cm/ Bottom Diameter 10.9 cm/ Height 33.3 cm/ Belly Depth 19.5 cm/ Weight 2,600 g

细长颈，中部微束，盘口，口边沿上卷，鼓腹，腹部上束下敛，平底，肩有半圆形四系耳，腹部有弦纹。盛液体的容器。

广东中医药博物馆藏

The pot is designed with a thin and long neck which narrows down in the middle, a plate-shaped mouth with a scrolling rim, a drum abdomen contracted downwards, and a flat bottom. With four semi-circular handles on the shoulder and string patterns around the belly, the pot was utilized as a liquid container.

Preserved in Guangdong Chinese Medicine Museum

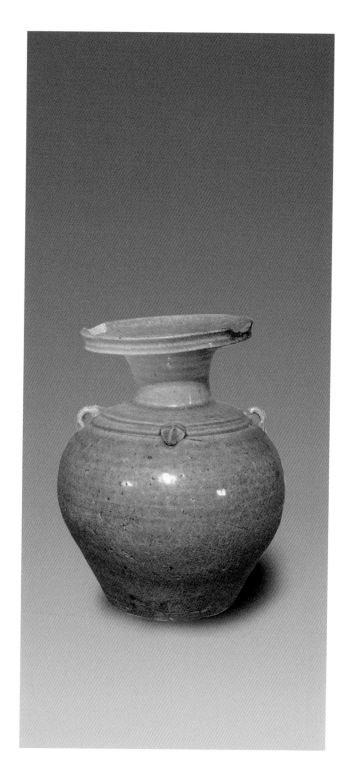

青瓷两系壶

晋

瓷质

腹径 17 厘米，高 20 厘米

Celadon Pot with Double Rings

Jin Dynasty

Porcelain

Belly Diameter 17 cm/ Height 20 cm

长颈，底部微束。盘口，口边缘上卷，微残。

鼓腹，平底，肩有半圆形四系耳。

广东中医药博物馆藏

With a long neck, a slightly tapered bottom, a plate-shaped mouth with the broken rim scrolling upwards, the pot has a drum belly, a flat bottom, and four semi-circular ears on the shoulder.

Preserved in Guangdong Chinese Medicine Museum

華

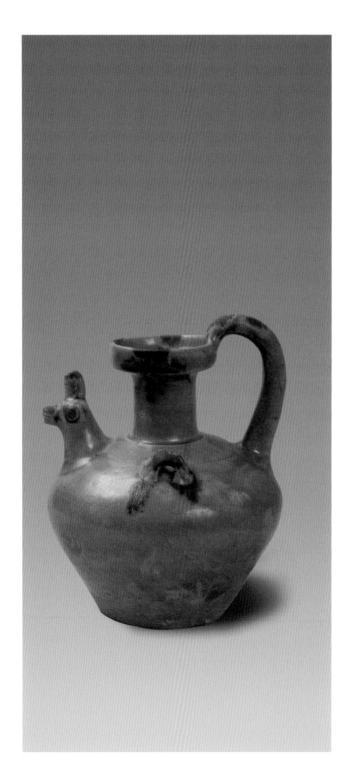

青釉褐斑瓷鸡首壶

东晋

瓷质

口径 5 厘米，底径 6 厘米，高 14 厘米

Celadon Ewer with Chicken-head Spout and Brown Speckles

Eastern Jin Dynasty

Porcelain

Mouth Diameter 5 cm/ Bottom Diameter 6 cm/

Height 14 cm

盘口，细颈，圆肩，鼓腹，中腰以下内收，平底。肩饰对称圆系，一端饰鸡首，引颈高冠，喙作流口，另一端作圆环形柄。肩身饰一道弦纹。灰白胎，施青绿色釉不到底，缀褐釉彩斑，自然而有层次感，与青色釉面相衬，分外和谐悦目。

南京博物院藏

The Ewer is designed with a plate-shaped mouth, a thin neck, a round shoulder, and a drum abdomen narrowing down from the waistline to the flat bottom. Circular ears symmetrically decorate the shoulder. One side of the shoulder is decorated with a chicken head with a craning neck, a long crest and a beak spout, while the other side a circular handle. The shoulder is incised with a line of string patterns, and the body is in pale grey. Except the bottom, the ewer is coated with dark green glaze embellished with brown-glazed speckles, which fit with the green glaze perfectly, providing the ewer with a sense of harmony and making it pleasing to the eye.

Preserved in Nanjing Museum

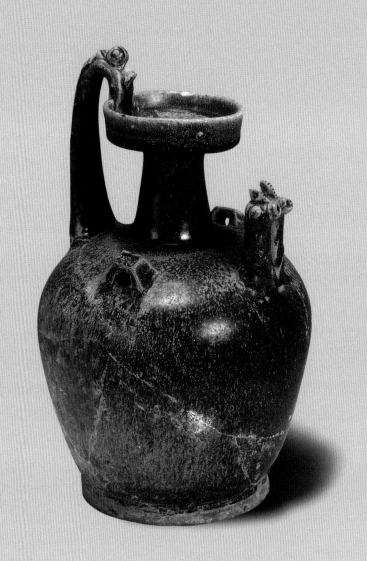

酱釉双鸡首壶

东晋

瓷质

口径 8.6 厘米，底径 11.8 厘米，高 26.6 厘米

Brown-glazed Ewer with Double Chicken-head Spout

Eastern Jin Dynasty

Porcelain

Mouth Diameter 8.6 cm/ Bottom Diameter 11.8 cm/ Height 26.6 cm

小盘口，细颈，肩部置对称方桥形横系。前置双鸡首，鸡圆嘴，高冠，长颈；后为双圆泥条形鋬，鋬上端塑龙首，龙口衔盘口沿，通体施酱色釉不及底。此器造型生动别致，为鸡首壶中之精品。1970年扬州市西湖乡平山村出土。

扬州博物馆藏

This ewer has a small flared-mouth and a thin neck. Two horizontal ears in the shape of a cubed bridge are symmetrically attached to its shoulder. In the front of the ewer are double chicken heads with a round mouth, a high crest and a long neck, while at the rear is a handle made of double circular clay strips. On the top of the handle is moulded a dragon head with the mouth holding the rim of the ewer. The ewer is covered with brown glaze except the base. With the vivid image and unique shape, it is an exquisite ewer with chicken-head spout. The ewer was excavated from Pingshan Village at West Lake Township in Yangzhou City, Jiangsu Province, in the year 1970.
Preserved in Yangzhou Museum

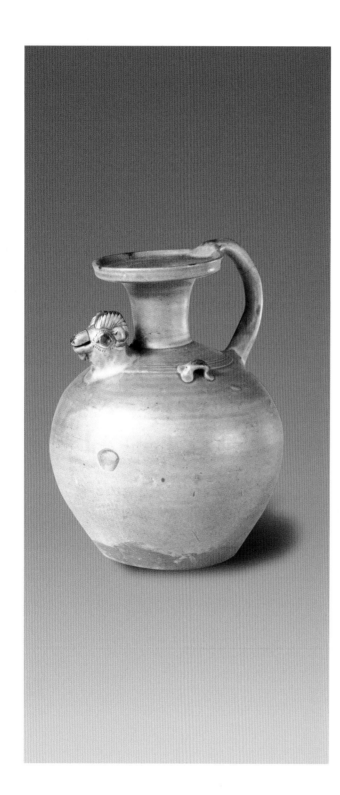

青釉羊首壶

东晋

瓷质

口径 10.8 厘米，足径 10.8 厘米，高 23.8 厘米

Celadon Ewer with Goat-head Spout

Eastern Jin Dynasty

Porcelain

Mouth Diameter 10.8 cm/ Foot Diameter 10.8 cm/

Height 23.8 cm

壶体洗口，细颈硕腹，肩与底径长度相若，平底。壶肩部凸起羊首形流，与流相对处置曲柄，柄连于口肩之间，另两面各有一横系，肩部画弦纹两道。通体施青釉，口沿、羊眼、系等处均饰以褐色斑点。

故宫博物院藏

The ewer is designed with a flared mouth, a thin neck, a big belly and a shoulder whose Diameter equals that of the flat bottom. A goat-head spout is attached to the sloping shoulder, opposite which is a curved handle, connecting the mouth and the shoulder. Horizontal rings are located at the other two sides of the shoulder with two lines of string patterns on it. Fully glazed with celadon, the ewer is embellished with brown speckles on the rim, the goat's eyes, and the rings as well.

Preserved in the Palace Museum

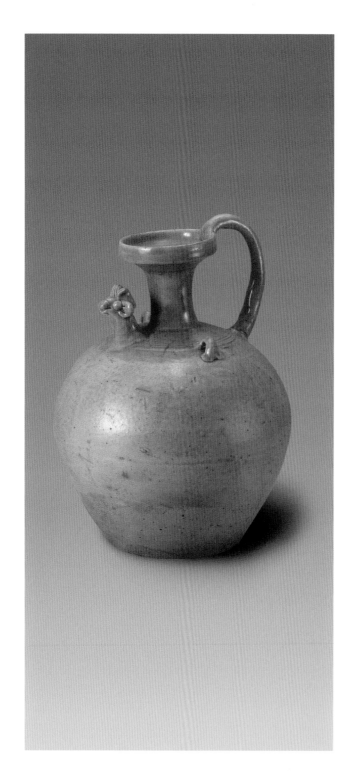

青釉羊首壶

东晋

瓷质

口径 9.1 厘米，底径 12.9 厘米，高 29.6 厘米

Celadon Ewer with Goat-head Spout

Eastern Jin Dynasty

Porcelain

Mouth Diameter 9.1 cm/ Bottom Diameter

12.9 cm/ Height 29.6 cm

小盘口，细颈，球腹，内凹底。肩部饰三道弦纹，两侧置对称条形竖系。前置一实心羊首，羊昂首，突目，卷角，后为条形鋬。通体施青灰色釉，施釉不及底，釉色均匀明亮。此器脱胎于当时流行的鸡首壶，羊首造型新颖独特。1985年邗江区甘泉乡六里村出土。

扬州博物馆藏

The ewer has a small flared mouth, a thin neck, a globular body and an inwardly concaved bottom with its shoulder decorated with string patterns. Strip-shaped vertical rings are placed on both sides of the shoulder. At the front end of the ewer is moulded a solid lifted goat head with the eyes embossed and horns curved, while at the rear is a strip-shaped handle. Except the bottom, the ewer is uniformly glazed with bright celadon. With the innovative design of a goat head, the vessel is born out of the popular ewer with a chicken-head spout at that time. It was unearthed from Six Mile Village at Ganquan Township in Hanjiang District, Jiangsu Province, in the year 1985.

Preserved in Yangzhou Museum

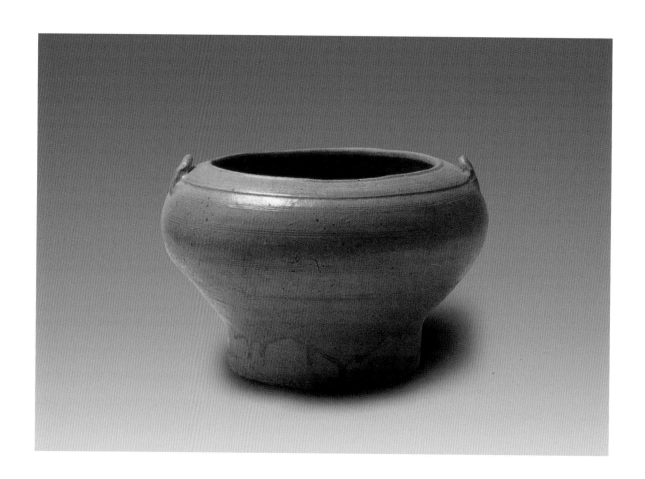

大口高足青瓷双耳罐

三国吴—西晋

瓷质

口径 18 厘米，腹径 26.8 厘米，底径 16 厘米，高 17 厘米

Green-glazed High-footed Jar with Double Ears

Three Kingdoms Period (Wu State) to Western Jin Dynasty

Porcelain

Mouth Diameter 18 cm/ Belly Diameter 26.8 cm/ Bottom Diameter 16 cm/ Height 17 cm

敛口，丰肩，圆腹渐收，直高足，淡青釉，施
釉不到底且有流釉现象，口沿微高，下饰一周
紧密细弦纹。肩上一对小桥形系，高出罐口，
罐身饰四道划纹，每道由三圈细凹弦纹组成。
平底，灰白胎，造型奇特。南京东郊甘家巷出土。

南京博物院藏

The vessel is designed with a contracted mouth,
a flattened shoulder and a swollen abdomen
narrowing down to the straight high-foot. It
is coated with a light greenish glaze running
downward to the bottom. The part below the
increasingly high rim is compactly decorated
with thin string patterns. On the shoulder of the
jar is a pair of small bridge-shaped ears, higher
than the rim. There are four lines incised on
the body, each of which is composed of three
fine grooves. With the body in pale grey, the
flat-bottomed jar stands out in shape. It was
unearthed from Ganjia Lane in the eastern
suburbs of Nanjing, Jiangsu Province.

Preserved in Nanjing Museum

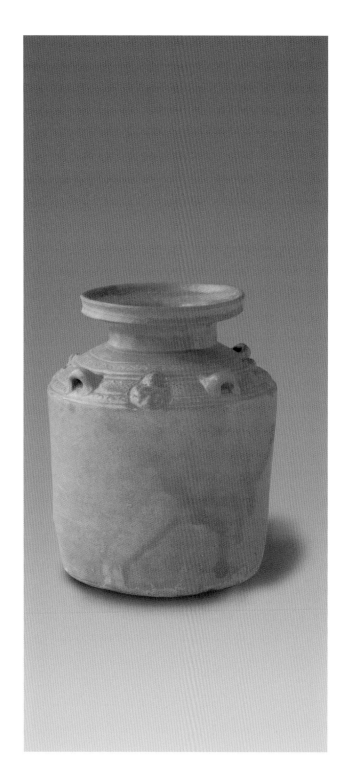

佛像贴塑青瓷四系盘口罐

西晋

瓷质

口径 10.5 厘米，底径 13 厘米，通高 17 厘米

Four-ringed Celadon Jar with Plate-shaped Mouth and Applique Buddha Images

Western Jin Dynasty

Porcelain

Mouth Diameter 10.5 cm/ Bottom Diameter 13 cm/

Height 17 cm

盘口，矮颈，斜肩微弧，直腹，平底，肩置四

个横向条形单系。肩部饰弦纹、纲格纹及系珠纹，

并堆贴四尊佛像。

南京浦口区文管会藏

The jar has a plate-shaped mouth, a short neck, a
sloping and slightly cambered shoulder, a straight
abdomen and a flat bottom. Four horizontal
single-strip handles are attached to the shoulder,
decorated with string patterns, grid patterns, and
bead motifs. Four appliqué Buddha images are
embossed on the shoulder too.

Preserved in the Department of Cultural Relics
Conservation of Pukou District in Nanjing City

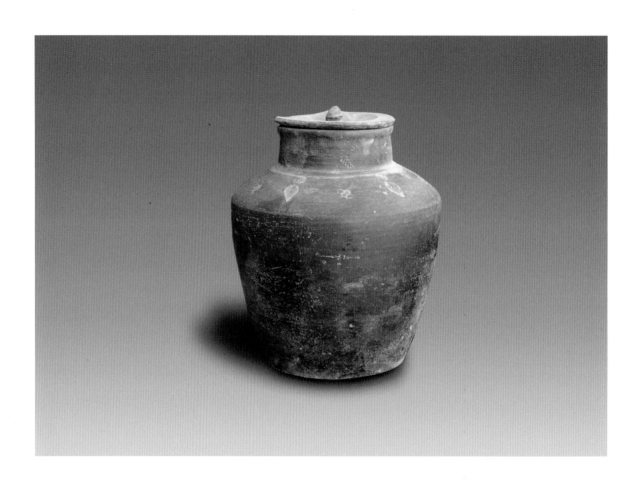

带盖灰陶罐

陶质

口径 11.7 厘米，底径 14 厘米，高 25 厘米，重 2000 克

Dark Grey Jar with Lid

Pottery

Mouth Diameter 11.7 cm/ Bottom Diameter 14 cm/ Height 25 cm/ Weight 2,000 g

直口，折肩，直斜腹，平底，黑陶，带一盖，
肩部有花卉图案。盛贮器。盖残。

陕西医史博物馆藏

The jar is a black pottery storage vessel with a
straight mouth, an angular shoulder, an oblique
vertical abdomen, a flat bottom and a lid. The
shoulder is decorated with floral motifs. The lid
is cracked.

Preserved in Shaanxi Museum of Medical History

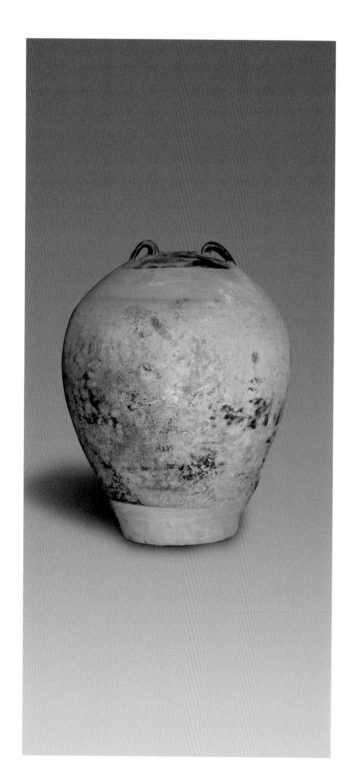

双耳带釉陶罐

陶质

口径 10.1 厘米，底径 11.3 厘米，高 25 厘米，

重 2900 克

Glazed Jar with Double Ears

Pottery

Mouth Diameter 10.1 cm/ Bottom Diameter

11.3 cm/ Height 25 cm/ Weight 2,900 g

圆肩，圆腹，圈足，肩部有两耳。肩、底无釉，

口、腹黑釉，罐内有粟。生活器具。口残。陕

西省澄城县征集。

陕西医史博物馆藏

The pottery jar, with the mouth damaged, has

a circular shoulder, a round belly and a ring

foot. There are two ears on both sides of the

shoulder. Both the shoulder and bottom are

unglazed, while the mouth and belly are glazed

black. Millets are found inside the jar. It was

used as a household utensil, and was collected

from Chengcheng County, Shaanxi Province.

Preserved in Shaanxi Museum of Medical History

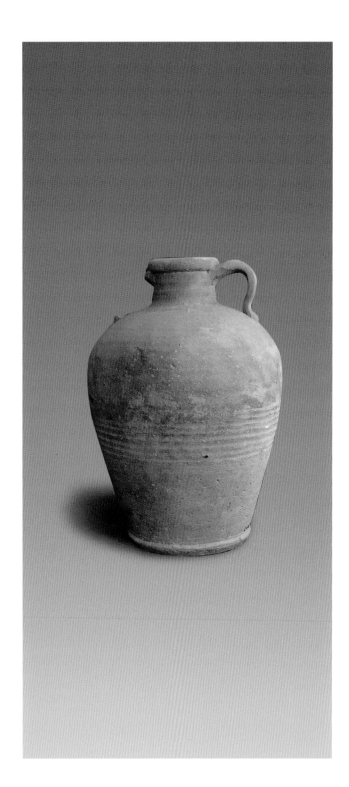

双耳陶罐

陶质

口径 11 厘米，底径 18 厘米，高 42 厘米，
重 6700 克

Double-eared Pottery Jar

Pottery

Mouth Diameter 11 cm/ Bottom Diameter 18 cm/

Height 42 cm/ Weight 6,700 g

唇口，直颈，圆肩，斜腹，浅圈足，腹部有数
道弦纹。盛贮器。一耳残。陕西省澄城县征集。

陕西医史博物馆藏

This pottery jar has a lip-shaped mouth rim, a
straight neck, a round shoulder, an oblique belly
with some string motifs on the surface, and a
shallow ring foot. This storage utensil with one
ear broken was collected from Chengcheng
County, Shaanxi Province.

Preserved in Shaanxi Museum of Medical History

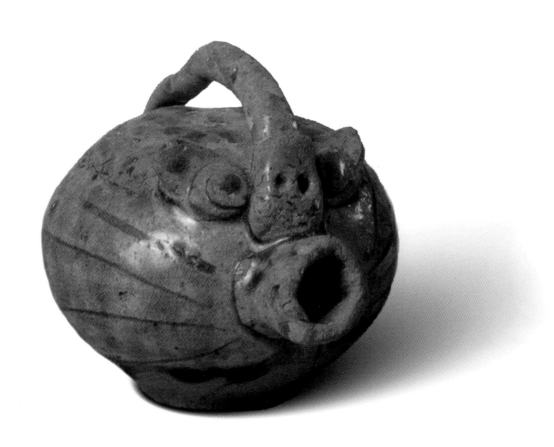

青釉猪形提梁注

东晋

瓷质

腹径 7.5 厘米，长 9 厘米，高 7.5 厘米

Swine-shaped Celadon Water Jet with Hoop Handle

Eastern Jin Dynasty

Porcelain

Belly Diameter 7.5 cm/ Length 9 cm/ Height 7.5 cm

灰胎，青黄釉，注形扁圆，腹空，壁侧塑一筒形注口作嘴，其上贴塑猪耳，一根带状提梁前接注口，戳孔作鼻，后接器背作尾，腹壁两侧有刻划纹。小猪造型生动，富有情趣。实用与装饰相结合的青瓷精品。

南京博物院藏

This water jet with a hoop handle has a grey body coated with greenish yellow glaze. It is characterized by an empty stomach, a cylindric spout with two swine-shaped ears attached to it, and a belt-shaped handle connecting the front spout and the back of the jet. The hoop handle has two holes as the pig's nose at the front and the rear is in the form of a tail. Both sides of the abdominal wall are decorated with incised lincs. The modelling of the swine is vivid and interesting. It is one of the most exquisite celadon jets both of functional and aesthetic value.

Preserved in Nanjing Museum

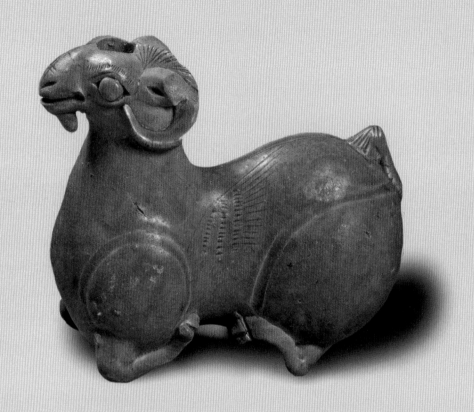

青釉羊形瓷水注

东晋

瓷质

长 15.5 厘米，高 12.4 厘米

Goat-shaped Celadon Water Jet

Eastern Jin Dynasty

Porcelain

Length 15.5 cm/ Height 12.4 cm

羊形，器身加点褐彩。颌下有须，项脊分披鬃毛，腹两侧刻画羽翼。四足曲于腹下作卧状，尾呈蕉叶状。青灰色胎，满施茶绿色釉，釉质润亮。造型生动，神态安详自如，给人一种典雅宁静的感觉，既是实用器，又是精美的瓷雕作品。南京新民门外象山七号墓出土。

南京博物院藏

The celadon water jet is shaped like a goat glazed with brown speckles. There is beard under the goat's chin, the ridge covered with bristles, and wings incised on both sides of its abdomen. The goat takes on a crouching posture with its knees bent down and its tail in the shape of banana leaves. The water jet has a grey body coated with glossy tea-greenish glaze. The vivid design and serene posture of the goat leaves an overall impression of elegance and tranquility. It is not only a functional household utensil, but also an exquisite example of porcelain carving works. It was excavated in the seventh tomb of Xiangshan Mountain at Xinmin Gate of Nanjing, Jiangsu Province.

Preserved in Nanjing Museum

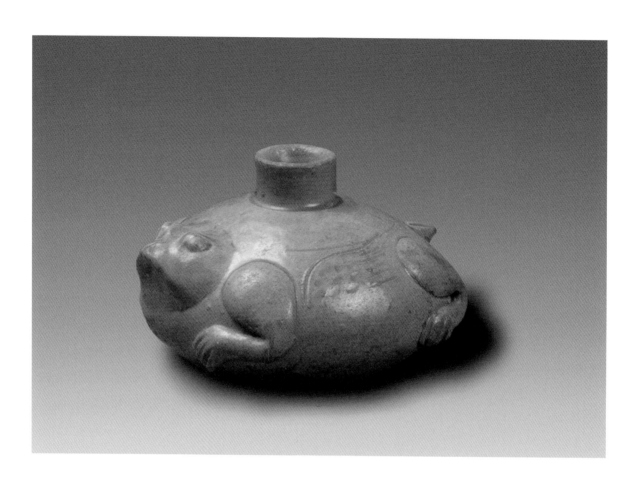

青瓷蛙形水盂

西晋

瓷质

口径 2.0 厘米，底径 3.9 厘米，高 5.4 厘米

Frog-shaped Celadon Water Jar

Western Jin Dynasty

Porcelain

Mouth Diameter 2.0 cm/ Bottom Diameter 3.9 cm/ Height 5.4 cm

浅灰色胎，淡绿釉，施釉不及底。蛙身为盂形，背上有一直筒流，头部和四肢采用模印贴塑手法，身后捏塑一小尾，蛙身两侧刻画出羽翼。整个造型如同一只正在水中游动的青蛙，极为生动。南京中华门外共青团路出土。

南京博物院藏

This water jar has a pale grey body covered with light greenish glaze and its bottom is unglazed. The jar is upside-down trumpet-shaped with its body in the shape of a frog, on the back of which stands a straight cylinder. The frog's head and four limbs are press moulded on the jar with a tiny kneaded tail and two wings incised on both sides of the frog body. An extremely vivid swimming frog is depicted by the design. It was excavated from Gongqingtuan Road, outside Zhonghua Gate of Nanjing, Jiangsu Province.

Preserved in Nanjing Museum

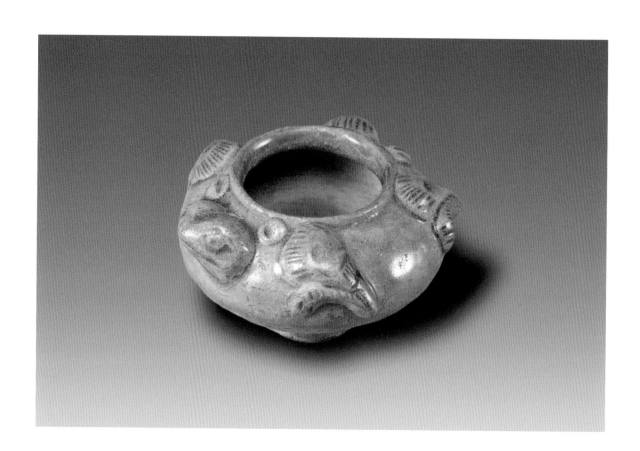

越窑青釉蛙形水盂

西晋

瓷质

口径 4 厘米，底径 3.2 厘米，高 3.6 厘米

Frog-shaped Celadon Water Jar, Yue Kiln

Western Jin Dynasty

Porcelain

Mouth Diameter 4 cm/ Bottom Diameter 3.2 cm/ Height 3.6 cm

直口，扁鼓腹，饼形足。腹部贴塑蛙的头、四足及尾。釉色青灰中泛黄，釉面开细纹片，足部无釉，露胎处呈灰褐色。

常州博物馆藏

This water jar has a straight mouth, a flat swelling belly with the head, limbs and tail of a frog moulded on it, and a pie-shaped foot. It is coated with yellowish green crackle glaze except for the foot which is unglazed. The body exposed is in greyish brown.

Preserved in Changzhou Museum

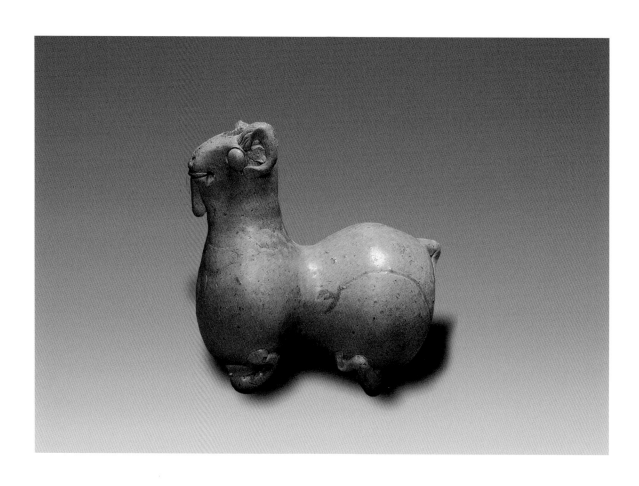

青瓷羊尊

东晋

瓷质

长 16.5 厘米，高 15 厘米

Goat-shaped Celadon Zun Vessel

Eastern Jin Dynasty

Porcelain

Length 16.5 cm/ Height 15 cm

釉呈青绿色，莹润不开片，胎色灰，胎釉烧结紧密，没有剥釉。贴塑双角绕于耳前，头顶有直径 1.5 厘米圆孔，双眼圆睁，颌下有须，舌头微露。脊上阴刻长线，身壮体肥。短尾，四足呈跪伏状，静卧安详，温驯可爱。堪称六朝早期青瓷器中的精品。南京市建邺路南侧建筑工地出土。

南京博物院藏

This bluish-green glazed Zun vessel is smooth and lustrous with uncracked glaze. The grey body is tightly glazed with no scalding. Two horns are windingly stamped before the goat's ears and a circular hole with a Diameter of 1.5 cm locates above its head. The goat has two round eyes, with beard under the chin, a slightly open mouth in which the tongue can be seen.and a short tail. A long line is incised on the ridge of this strong and plump goat. This gentle and lovely goat takes on a crouching posture with its knees bent down in a quiet and peaceful manner. It can be regarded as an exquisite piece of celadon ware in the early Six Dynasties. It was excavated from a construction site in the south of Jianye Road, Nanjing, Jiangsu Province.

Preserved in Nanjing Museum

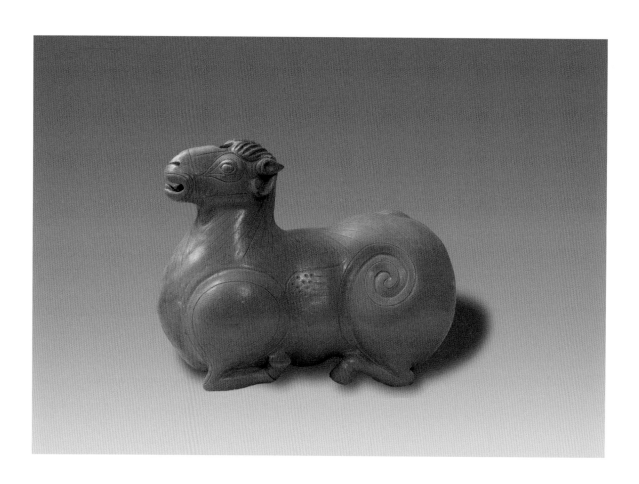

青瓷羊尊

西晋

瓷质

长 26 厘米，高 20.3 厘米

Goat-shaped Celadon Zun Vessel

Western Jin Dynasty

Porcelain

Length 26 cm/ Height 20.3 cm

平首，作瞪目远视状，张口，竖耳，双角后卷，体壮硕，腹两侧刻画出羽翼，四足屈于腹下作卧伏态。头顶有一圆孔，空腹。造型生动，神态祥和安谧，给人典雅神秘之美。南京西岗西晋墓出土。

南京博物院藏

This celadon Zun vessel is in the shape of a chubby goat with a flat head, round eyes seemingly looking afar, an open mouth, erected ears and two backward curving horns. Two wings are incised on both sides of the stomach, under which four limbs are buckling. The goat takes on a crouching posture. There is a circular hole on the top of its head and the stomach is hollow in side. The vivid design and tranquil expression display a kind of elegant and mysterious beauty. It was excavated from a tomb of the Western Jin Dynasty in Xigang District, Nanjing, Jiangsu Province.
Preserved in Nanjing Museum

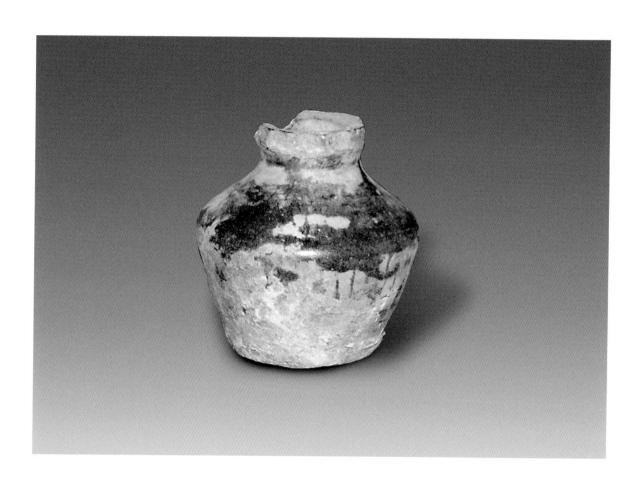

釉小陶瓶

陶质

口径 2.7 厘米，底径 3.5 厘米，高 5.4 厘米，重 100 克

Small Glazed Jar

Pottery

Mouth Diameter 2.7 cm/ Bottom Diameter 3.5 cm/ Height 5.4 cm/ Weight 100 g

侈口，斜肩，斜腹，圈足，足部无釉，棕釉。生活器具。口沿残。陕西省澄城县征集。

陕西医史博物馆藏

This brown-glazed jar is characterized by a wide flared mouth, a sloping shoulder, an oblique belly and an unglazed ring foot. This household utensil with a broken mouth rim was collected from Chengcheng County, Shaanxi Province.

Preserved in Shaanxi Museum of Medical History

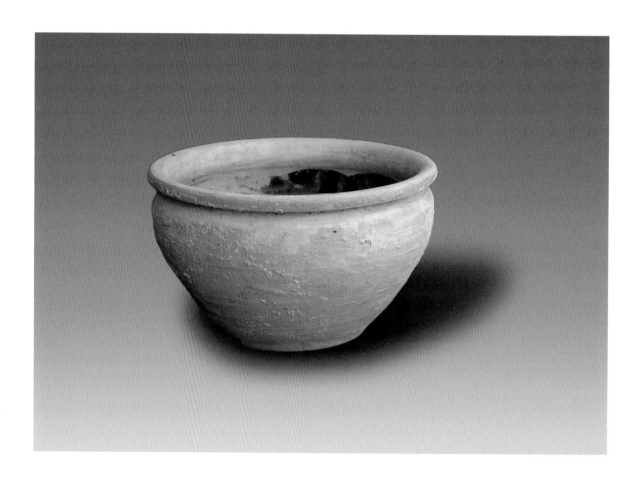

陶盆

陶质

口径 20.5 厘米，底径 11.2 厘米，高 13 厘米，重 1300 克

Pottery Basin

Pottery

Mouth Diameter 20.5 cm/ Bottom Diameter 11.2 cm/ Height 13 cm/ Weight 1,300 g

圆唇，斜腹，浅圈足，盆内施黑釉。盛贮器。

完整无损。陕西省澄城县征集。

陕西医史博物馆藏

This basin is characterized by a round lip, an oblique belly, a shallow ring foot and black glazed interior. This intact storage utensil was collected from Chengcheng County, Shaanxi Province.

Preserved in Shaanxi Museum of Medical History

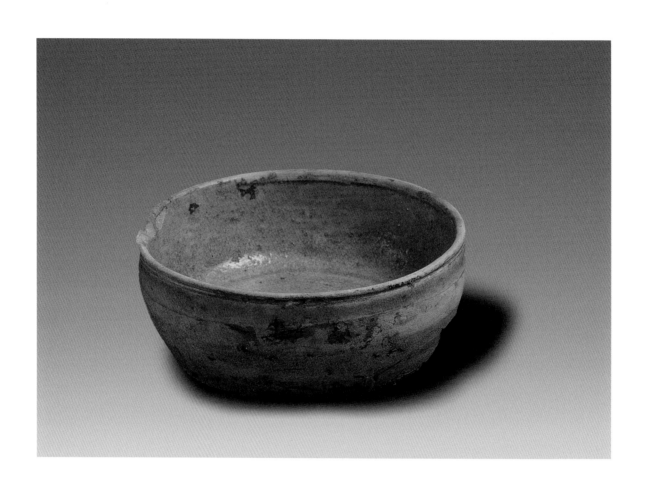

墨书"谢"字款瓷钵

东晋

瓷质

口径 15 厘米，底径 12.5 厘米，高 6 厘米

Bowl Inked with Chinese Character "Xie"

Eastern Jin Dynasty

Porcelain

Mouth Diameter 15 cm/ Bottom Diameter 12.5 cm/ Height 6 cm

圆唇，直口微敞，弧腹，平底。外壁口沿下方
饰凹弦纹带。黄白胎，施黄绿色釉。外底有一
墨书"谢"字，书法中含内敛，颇具晋人风范。
该器出土于秦淮河来燕桥南侧古乌衣巷地下约
6米处的六朝地层内，对研究东晋王谢家族与
乌衣巷的关系有重要意义。

南京王谢古居陈列馆藏

This bowl has a round rim, a slightly flared
straight mouth, a cambered belly and a flat foot.
The outer wall below the mouth rim is decorated
with bands of concaving string pattern. Its
yellow and white body is glazed yellowish
green. Inked at the exterior bottom is a Chinese
character "Xie", written in a restrained style,
which is quite similar to the calligraphic style in
the Jin Dynasty. This object was excavated from
the underground stratum of the Six Dynasties,
about 6 meters under the ancient Wuyi (Black
Clothes) Lane, to the south of Laiyan Bridge,
Qinhuai River. It is of great significance for the
researches on Wuyi Lane (Wang's and Xie's
old residences) and the relations between the
influential families—Wang and Xie.
Preserved in the Exhibition Hall of Former
Residence of Wang Xie in Nanjing

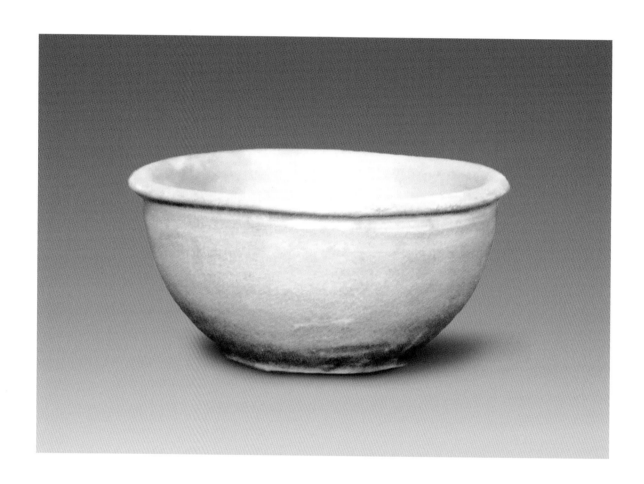

黄釉瓷碗

晋

瓷质

口径 17 厘米，高 6.5 厘米

Yellow-glazed Bowl

Jin Dynasty

Porcelain

Mouth Diameter 17 cm/ Height 6.5 cm

碗状，口沿外折，鼓腹，圈足，施黄釉。造型精致，朴实，浑厚。

广东中医药博物馆藏

With everted rim, the yellow-glazed bowl has a round belly and a ring foot, demonstrating an exquisite design and neat structure.

Preserved in Guangdong Chinese Medicine Museum

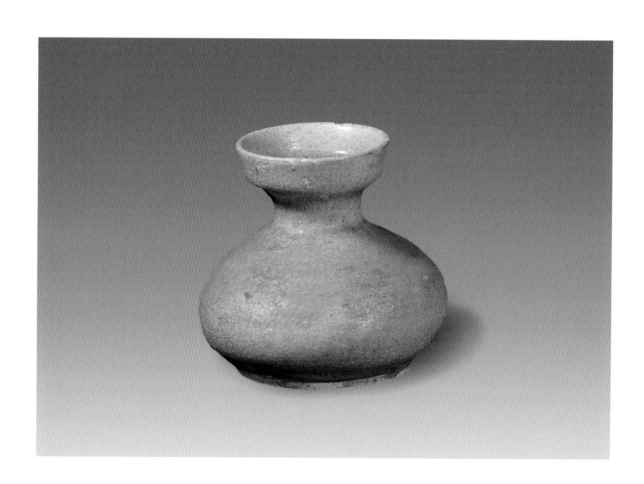

青瓷唾壶

晋

瓷质

口径 7.8 厘米，底径 9 厘米，高 11.8 厘米

Celadon Spittoon

Jin Dynasty

Porcelain

Mouth Diameter 7.8 cm/ Bottom 9 cm/ Height 11.8 cm

深盘口，短颈，斜肩，垂腹，圈足。系南京栖
霞山甘家巷化肥厂出土。

南京博物院藏

The spittoon has a deep plate-shaped mouth,
a short neck, a sloping shoulder, a vertical
belly and a ring foot. It was excavated from a
chemical fertilizer plant at Ganjia Lane, Qixia
Mountain in Nanjing, Jiangsu Province.
Preserved in Nanjing Museum

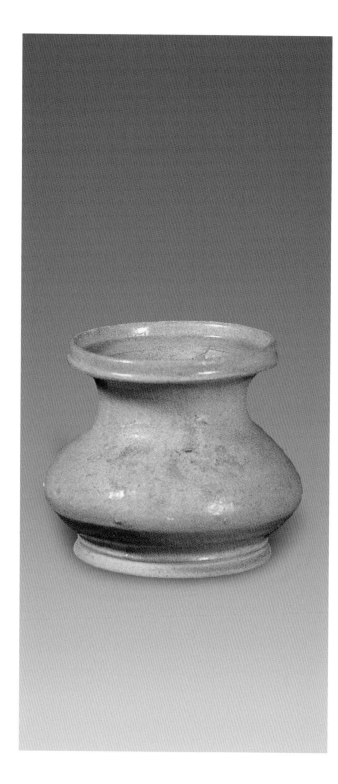

青瓷唾壶

晋

瓷质

口径 8 厘米，底径 7.5 厘米，高 8.3 厘米

Celadon Spittoon

Jin Dynasty

Porcelain

Mouth Diameter 8 cm/ Bottom Diameter 7.5 cm/

Height 8.3 cm

盘口，短颈，斜肩，鼓腹，圈足。西晋元康三
年（293）制。南京中华门郎家山出土。

南京博物院藏

The spittoon is featured with a dish-shaped
mouth, a short neck, a sloping shoulder, a drum
abdomen and a ring foot. It was made in the
third year of Yuankang Period of the Western
Jin Dynasty and excavated from Langjia
Mountain at the Zhonghua Gate of Nanjing,
Jiangsu Province.

Preserved in Nanjing Museum

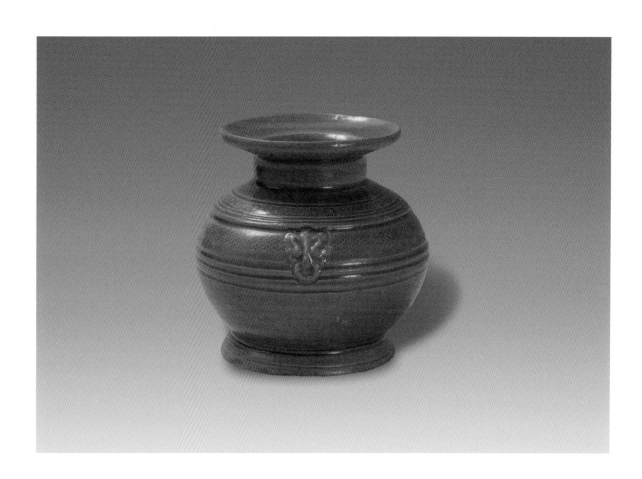

青釉印花唾壶

西晋

瓷质

口径 9.2 厘米，底径 9.3 厘米，高 11.5 厘米

Celadon Spittoon with Floral Designs

Western Jin Dynasty

Porcelain

Mouth Diameter 9.2 cm/ Bottom Diameter 9.3 cm/ Height 11.5 cm

胎灰白，质坚硬。盘口，短颈，鼓腹似球体，假圈足外撇，器形呈鱼篓形。肩部压印联珠纹，联珠纹上下各刻画多道弦纹。腹部压印一圈宽斜方格细纹，在斜方格上有距离相等的三个模印铺首。通体施青绿色釉，釉面光亮匀净。江苏省江宁县小丹阳镇出土。

南京博物院藏

This creel-shaped spittoon has a grey and white body and hard texture, with a plate mouth, a short neck, a globular sphere-like body, and a fake ring foot turning outward. Its shoulder is stamped with a motif of linked pearls, above and below which are incised many string patterns. A wide band of oblique and checkered patterns are stamped on the stomach, above which are pressed three equidistant animal head applique rings. The spittoon is fully celadon glazed with smooth luster. It was excavated from Xiaodanyang Town in Jiangning County, Jiangsu Province.

Preserved in Nanjing Museum

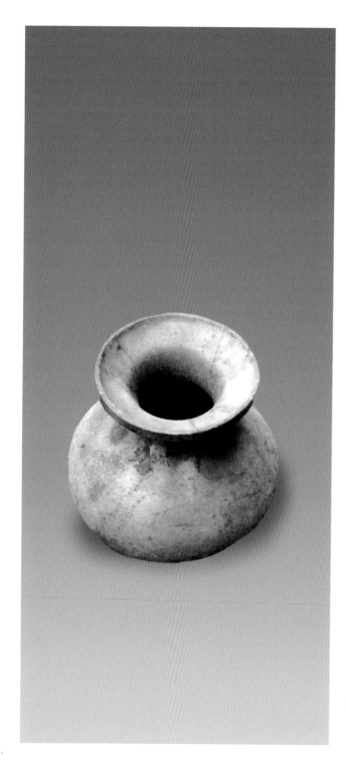

青瓷唾壶

晋

瓷质

上口径 9.5 厘米，底径 9.5 厘米，壶身直径
13.9 厘米，高 12.1 厘米，腹深 11 厘米

敞口，鼓腹，储容器。

广东中医药博物馆藏

Celadon Spittoon

Jin Dynasty

Porcelain

Upper Mouth Diameter 9.5 cm/ Bottom
Diameter 9.5 cm/ Body Diameter 13.9 cm/
Height 12.1 cm/ Depth 11 cm

This spittoon with a flared mouth and a
swelling belly was utilized as a container.

Preserved in Guangdong Chinese Medicine
Museum

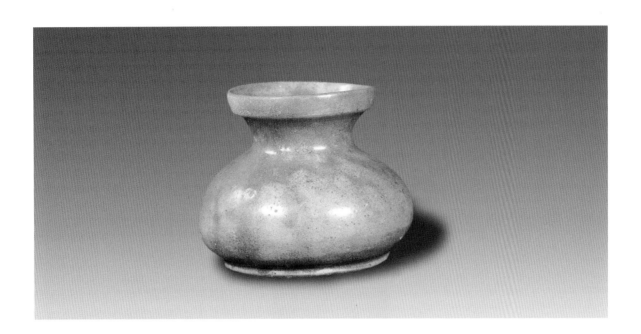

青瓷唾壶

晋

瓷质

口径 8.5 厘米，底径 10 厘米，高 10 厘米

假圈足，平底，外施以青黄色釉。

上海中医药博物馆藏

Celadon Spittoon

Jin Dynasty

Porcelain

Mouth Diameter 8.5 cm/ Bottom Diameter 10 cm/ Height 10 cm

The bottom of the spittoon is flat with a false ring foot. The whole spittoon is coated with greenish yellow glaze.

Preserved in Shanghai Museum of Traditional Chinese Medicine

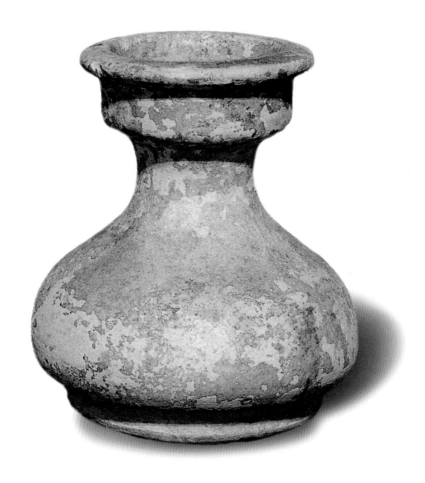

唾壶

晋

瓷质

腹径 15 厘米，高 20 厘米

深盘口，口沿外折，长颈，斜肩，垂腹，圈足。

造型精致，朴实，厚重。

广东中医药博物馆藏

Spittoon

Jin Dynasty

Porcelain

Belly Diameter 15 cm/ Height 20 cm

The spittoon was designed with a deep plate-shaped mouth with the rim scrolling outward, a long neck, a sloping shoulder, a vertical belly and a ring foot, reflecting a simple structure and exquisite workmanship.

Preserved in Guangdong Chinese Medicine Museum

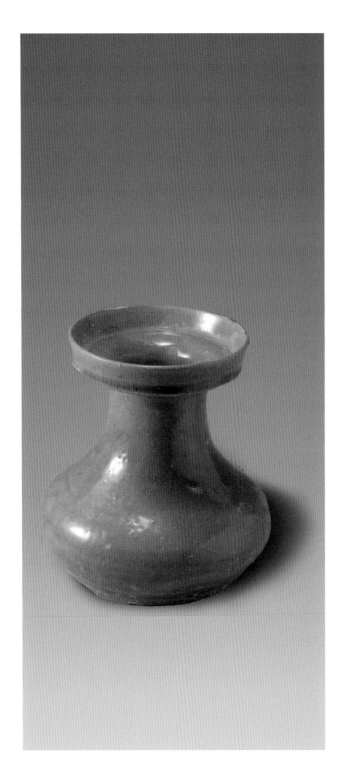

青瓷唾盂

东晋

瓷质

口径 4.4 厘米，腹径 6 厘米，高 12.6 厘米

Celadon Spittoon

Eastern Jin Dynasty

Porcelain

Mouth Diameter 4.4 cm/ Belly Diameter 6 cm/

Height 12.6 cm

盘口，长颈，斜肩，垂腹。1993 年上虞市小越镇新宅驮山出土。

浙江上虞区文物管理所藏

The plate-shaped spittoon has a long neck, a sloping shoulder and a straight belly. This spittoon was excavated from Tuo Mountain of Xin Zhai Village, Xiao Yue Town, Shangyu City, Zhejiang Province, in 1993.
Preserved in Department of Cultural Relics Conservation of Shangyu District, Zhejiang

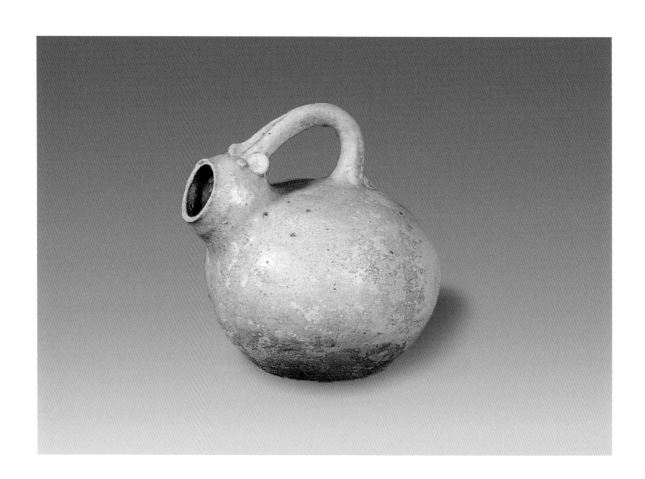

青瓷圆虎子

晋

瓷质

口径 5.3 厘米，底径 11.1 厘米，通高 20.5 厘米

Circular Celadon Holy Vase

Jin Dynasty

Porcelain

Mouth Diameter 5.3 cm/ Bottom Diameter 11.1 cm/ Height 20.5 cm

平底，圆腹，口端虎头形，双目圆瞪，把连接
口与器身，造型朴素。西晋太康四年（283）制。
江苏江宁区秣陵元塘出土。

南京博物院藏

With a glaring-eyed tiger head decorated on the
mouth, the vase has a flat bottom and a round
belly. The mouth of the vase is combined by the
handle with its body, reflecting a neat and bold
design. The vase was made in the year 283 A.D.
(the forth year of Taikang reign of the Western
Jin Dynasty). It was unearthed in Yuantang
Village of Moling Town, Jiangning District,
Jiangsu Province.

Preserved in Nanjing Museum

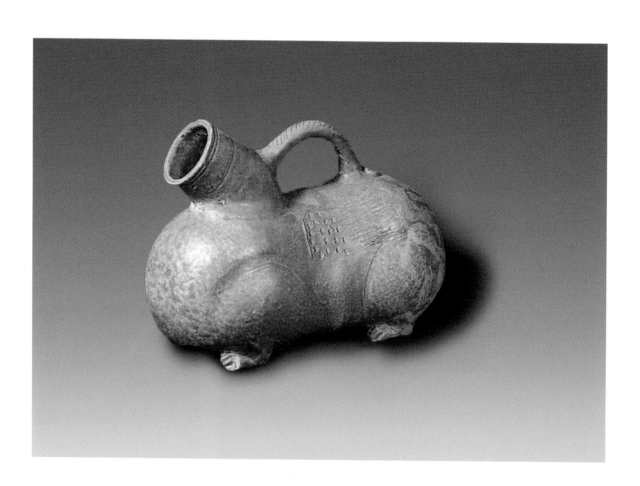

青瓷虎子

晋

瓷质

长 23.5 厘米，口径 5.7 厘米，高 18 厘米

Celadon Holy Vase

Jin Dynasty

Porcelain

Length 23.5 cm / Mouth Diameter 5.7 cm / Height 18 cm

体呈蚕茧形，圆口，背上有圆形细长提梁，提
梁末端贴有细小尾，两肋刻画双翼，下有蹲伏
四足。造型别致。西晋元康四年（294）制。
江苏句容市石狮公社孙西生产队汜年墓出土。

南京博物院藏

The holy vase was designed in a unique style
with a cocoon-shaped body, a round mouth,
a slender handle on its back, and a small tail
attached to the end of the handle. The side
wings are incised on the abdomen, with four
squatting feet molded at the bottom. This holy
vase was made in the year of 294 A.D. (the
4th year of Yuankang reign of the Western Jin
Dynasty). It was unearthed in Sinian Tomb in
the field of Sunxi Production Team of Shishi
Commune, Jurong City, Jiangsu Province.
Preserved in Nanjing Museum

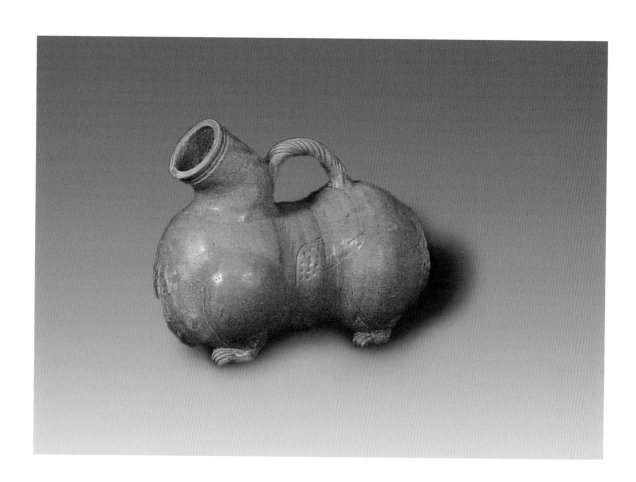

青瓷虎子

晋

瓷质

口径 6.4 厘米，长 23 厘米，高 19 厘米

Celadon Holy Vase

Jin Dynasty

Porcelain

Mouth Diameter 6.4 cm/ Length 23 cm/ Height 19 cm

体呈蚕茧形，圆口，背上有绳纹提梁，两肋刻画双翼，四足蹲曲。西晋时制。江苏六合区草塘公社彭凹大队出土。

南京博物院藏

The holy vase has a cocoon-shaped body, a round mouth, and four squatting feet. On the back there is a handle embellished with rope patterns, with side wings incised on the abdomen. This holy vase was made during the period of the Western Jin Dynasty. It was unearthed in the field of Peng'ao Production Team of Caotang Commune, Liuhe District, Jiangsu Province.

Preserved in Nanjing Museum

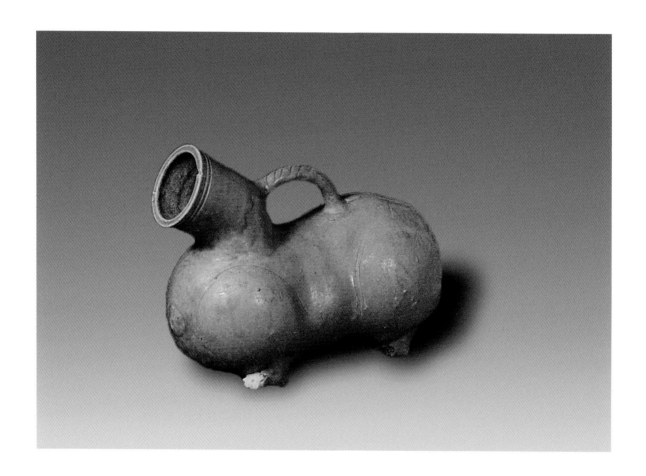

青瓷虎子

晋

瓷质

口径 5.7 厘米，长 21.8 厘米，高 18 厘米

Celadon Holy Vase

Jin Dynasty

Porcelain

Mouth Diameter 5.7 cm/ Length 21.8 cm/ Height 18 cm

体呈蚕茧形，圆口，背上有绳纹提梁，提梁连接口与器身，下有蹲伏四足。东吴时制。南京栖霞山甘家巷化肥厂出土。

南京博物院藏

The holy vase is featured with a cocoon-shaped body, a round mouth and four squatting feet at the lower part. A handle with rope patterns is on the back, connecting the mouth and the body. This holy vase was made during the period of the Eastern Wu Dynasty. It was unearthed in the fertilizer plant of Ganjia Lane, Qixia Mountain in Nanjing, Jiangsu Province.

Preserved in Nanjing Museum

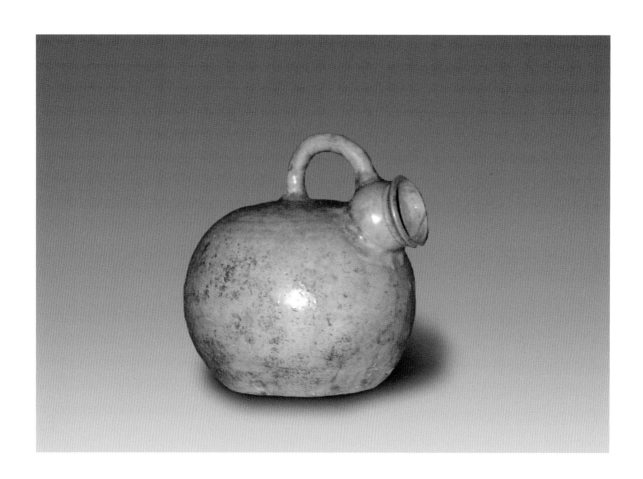

陶虎子

晋

陶质

口内径 4.15 厘米，口外径 6.15 厘米，通高 21.5 厘米

Pottery Holy Vase

Jin Dynasty

Pottery

Inner Diameter 4.15 cm/ Outer Diameter 6.15 cm/ Height 21.5 cm

该藏通身施土黄釉,有提梁,上部有口,工艺粗糙,
底部无款,无盖。壶形,为盛药器具。1955年入藏。
保存基本完好, 口有残。

中华医学会 / 上海中医药大学医史博物馆藏

The yellowish-brown-glazed holy vase has a
handle and a mouth on the upper part. This lidless
vase is rough in workmanship with no inscription
on the bottom. This pot-shaped vase was used as a
drug container. Collected in the year 1955, it has
been kept intact with just the mouth crackled.
Preserved in Chinese Medical Association/Museum of
Chinese Medicine, Shanghai University of Traditional
Chinese Medicine

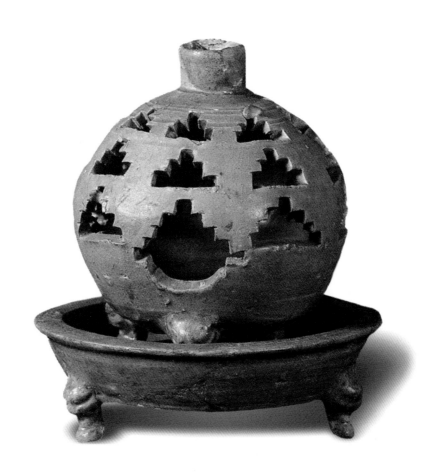

青瓷香熏

西晋

瓷质

盘口径 15.5 厘米，底径 12 厘米，通高 17 厘米

用于室内或服饰熏香，改善居室卫生和个人卫生。江苏无锡市东峰公社东方红大队张家湾生产队出土。

南京博物院藏

Celadon Censer

Western Jin Dynasty

Porcelain

Plate Mouth Diameter 15.5 cm/ Bottom Diameter 12 cm/ Height 17 cm

The censer is designed and made for the purpose of perfuming the room and clothing so as to improve room sanitation and personal hygiene. It was excavated in the field of Zhangjiawan production team belonging to Red East Production Brigade, Dongfeng Commune, Wuxi city in Jiangsu Province.

Preserved in Nanjing Museum

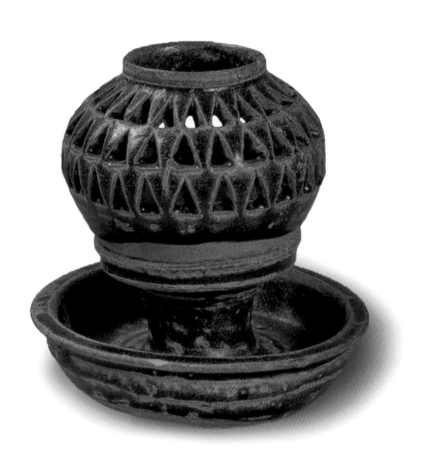

褐釉瓷香熏

东晋

瓷质

口径 5.2 厘米，高 11.2 厘米

Brown-glazed Pottery Censer

Eastern Jin Dynasty

Porcelain

Mouth Diameter 5.2 cm/ Height 11.2 cm

褐釉，由熏炉、承柱和承盘组成。上部熏炉为球形，敛口，圆唇，鼓腹，腹上满布三角形镂孔，分三行排列。承柱为圆柱形，较低矮，承盘口沿宽边，盘口处旋刻一周旋纹。通体施褐釉，色调深沉，反映了东晋时期青瓷发展已从青釉单一品种发展到其他品种。江宁陶吴镇娘娘山出土。

南京博物院藏

This brown-glazed censer has three parts: censing basket, bearing column and bearing basin. The censing basket on the upper part is in the shape of a sphere with a contracted mouth, a round rim and a globular body. The belly is covered with triangular engraved holes arrayed in three lines. The bearing column is short and cylinder-shaped while the basin has a broad rim, incised with string patterns. The whole censer is covered with brown glaze in dark tone, suggesting that the glaze range expanded during the Eastern Jin Dynasty and there were diverse glaze recipes instead of the earlier celadon glaze. It was excavated from Niangniang Mountain in Taowu County, Jiangning District.

Preserved in Nanjing Museum

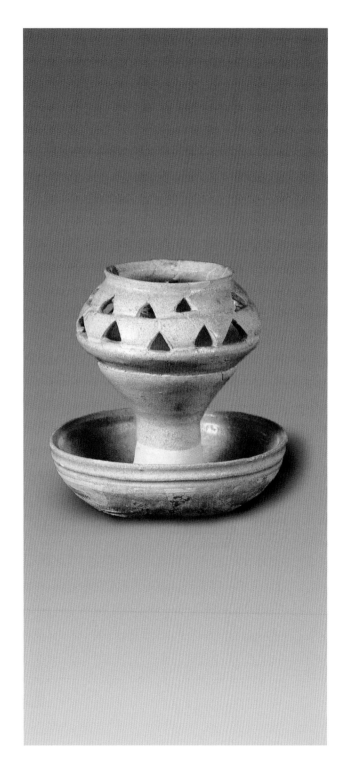

青瓷香熏

东晋

瓷质

通高 13.2 厘米

香笼：口径 7.5 厘米，腹深 5.4 厘米

盘：口径 13.8 厘米，底径 9.5 厘米

Celadon Censer

Eastern Jin Dynasty

Porcelain

Height 13.2 cm

Censer cage: Mouth Diameter 7.5 cm/ Depth 5.4 cm

Basin: Mouth Diameter 13.8 cm/ Bottom Diameter 9.5 cm

此器分为熏体与盘状底座。熏体上半部分有两排排列规则的三角形透雕烟孔，构成大小逐渐变化，造型典雅别致。南京光华门外赵士岗M10 墓出土。

南京博物院藏

This object is composed of an incense burner and a dish-shaped base. On the upper part of the burner, two rows of triangular ventholes, whose area decrease from the lower row to the upper row, were regularly pieced, displaying an elegant and unique design. It was excavated from the tenth mausoleum on Zhaoshi Hill outside Guanghua Gate of Nangjing City, Jiangsu Province.

Preserved in Nanjing Museum

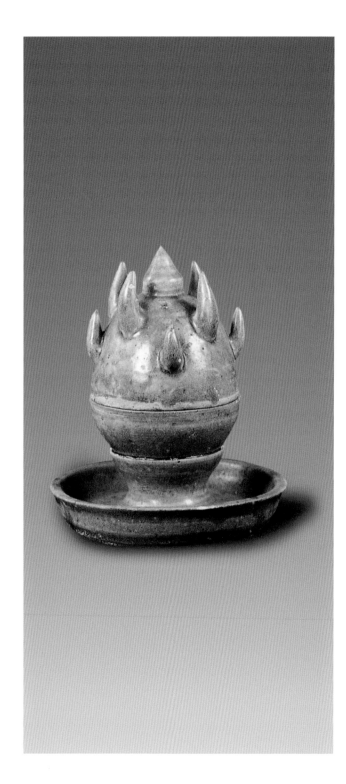

青瓷香熏

晋

瓷质

底径 11.5 厘米，通高 16 厘米

Celadon Censer

Jin Dynasty

Porcelain

Bottom Diameter 11.5 cm/ Height 16 cm

器物上尖角状物主要起支架作用，可熏帽用。

上海中医药博物馆藏

There are some pointed horns on the upper part of the censer, with a function of supporting a cap when being fumigated.

Preserved in Shanghai Museum of Traditional Chinese Medicine

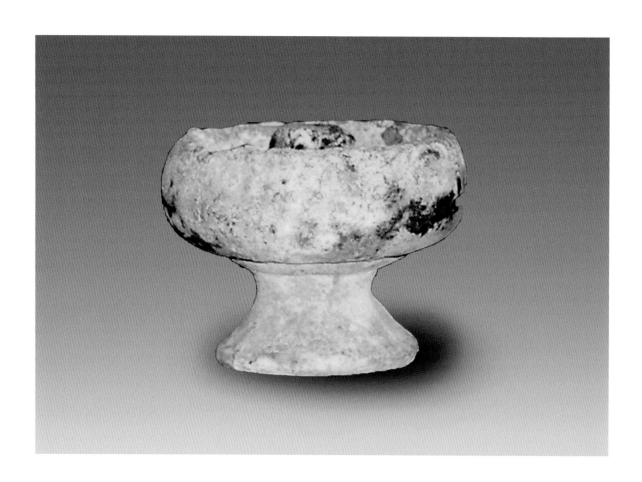

灯

瓷质

口径 6 厘米，底径 4 厘米，通高 4.5 厘米，重 150 克

Lamp

Porcelain

Mouth Diameter 6 cm/ Bottom Diameter 4 cm/ Height 4.5 cm/ Weight 150 g

束口，喇叭形底座，灯碗内有一柱眼，棕釉。

日用陶器。完整无损。

陕西医史博物馆藏

The lamp has a pedestal in the shape of a trumpet and a tapering mouth on the top. There is a brown-glazed pillar to support the lampwick in the lamp fire bowl. The lamp, designed for everyday use, is still in good shape.

Preserved in Shaanxi Museum of Medical History

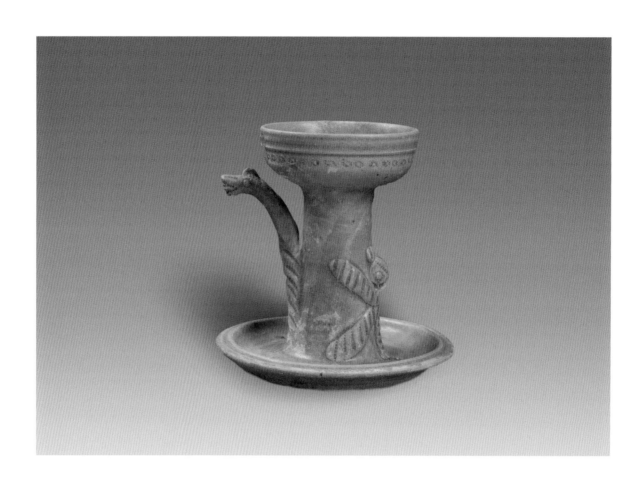

青釉龙柄瓷灯

西晋

瓷质

口径 9.9 厘米，高 15.2 厘米

Celadon Lamp with Dragon-shaped Handle

Western Jin Dynasty

Porcelain

Mouth Diameter 9.9 cm/ Height 15.2 cm

下部为宽沿平底的圆盘，盘沿上饰弦纹，盘中立一圆柱，柱上贴一熊首及四肢，熊两前爪支于两后爪之上，一前爪取食进口，一前爪抓耳挠痒，柱另一边贴一龙柄，龙微露齿，圆睁两目。灯柱上承一灯盏，盏外壁饰弦纹、联珠纹。此灯造型别致优雅，釉色洁净美观，集实用、观赏于一体，是一件十分珍贵的六朝青瓷精品。南京雨花台区丁墙村出土。

南京博物院藏

The lower part of the lamp is a broad-brimmed and flat-bottomed basin. Covered by string patterns on the rim, the basin has a bearing column in the middle, on which were pasted a bear's head and its four limbs. The bear's front paws are propped up on the rear ones. One front paw is snatching food, while the other is scratching the ear. To the opposite side of the column is attached a dragon-shaped handle. The dragon stares up with eyes wide open and teeth exposed. The lampstand supported by the bearing column is decorated with string patterns and a linked-pearl pattern. With elegant design and beautiful glaze, this lamp, an exquisite and valuable example of celadon ware made in the Six Dynasties, is of both functional and aesthetic values. It was excavated from Dingqiang Village of Yuhuatai District, Nanjing City.

Preserved in Nanjing Museum

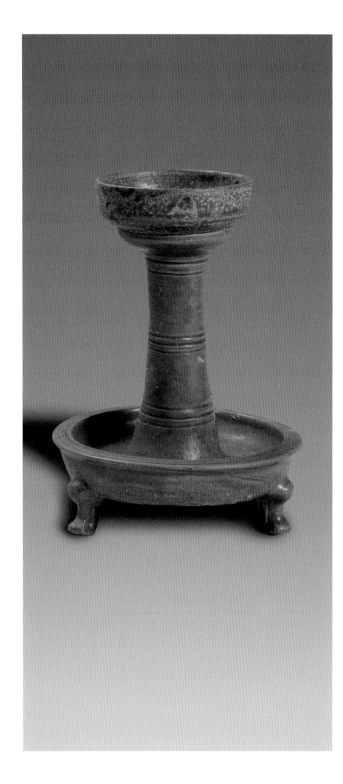

青瓷兽足灯

东晋

瓷质

高 24.3 厘米

Celadon Lamp with Paw-shaped Pedestal

Eastern Jin Dynasty

Porcelain

Height 24.3 cm

灯上部以小青瓷盏作灯盏，与上细下粗的高承柱相连，承柱上饰两组弦纹，下为有三个兽蹄足的圆形承盘。胎灰白，遍施青釉。其造型别致新颖，是古代青瓷灯具中少见的精品。南京象山七号墓出土。

南京博物院藏

The upper part of the lamp is a celadon lampstand supported by a tapering bearing column, surrounded with two bands of string patterns, under which is a circular basin with three stabilizer bars in the shape of beast hoofs. The celadon lamp is glazed with a greyish white body. Unconventional in pattern and unique in style, this lamp is exquisite and rare in the collection of ancient celadon lamps. It was excavated in No. 7 Tomb on Elephant Mountain, Nanjing City.

Preserved in Nanjing Museum

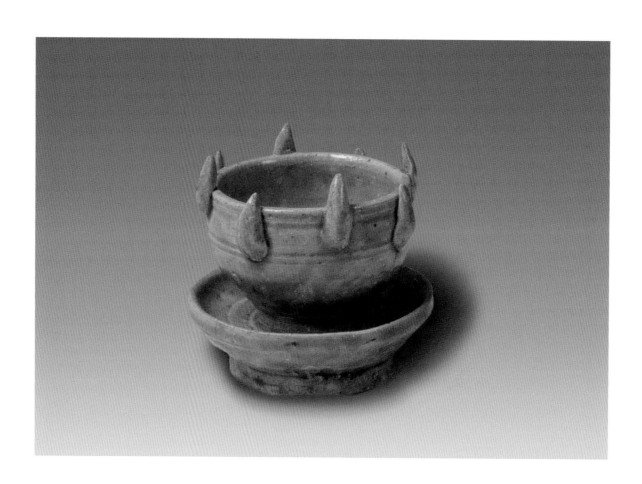

越窑青釉塑火焰形灯

晋

瓷质

口径 6.8 厘米，底径 5.6 厘米，通高 7.8 厘米

Celadon Flame-shaped Lamp, Yue Kiln

Jin Dynasty

Porcelain

Mouth Diameter 6.8 cm/ Bottom Diameter 5.6 cm/ Height 7.8 cm

平底，饼足微外撇，下盘口沿微内敛，盏敛口，深腹。外壁口沿及腹部各饰弦纹两道。口沿粘贴火焰形泥条八个，间距均等，四高四低，两两相对。胎质坚硬，呈灰白色。通体施釉不及底，釉质纯净，色调青翠。此器最引人注目的特征是灯盏口沿所饰的火焰塑形，用造型语言的象征意义，体现先民对火焰的崇拜和对光明的向往。

南京博物院藏

The pie-shaped foot of the lamp is slightly curved outward while the rim of the plate underneath is contracted. With a contracted mouth and a deep belly, the lamp holder is incised with two bands of string patterns around the rim and the belly. Eight equidistant flame-shaped clay-strips are arranged symmetrically, half of which are arrayed a little bit higher than the rest. The grey body is hard in texture. The fully applied celadon glaze is in pure verdant and stops above the bottom. The most notable feature of this lamp is the flame-shaped design at the mouth, embodying the ancient Chinese people's worship and yearning for flame and light.

Preserved in Nanjing Museum

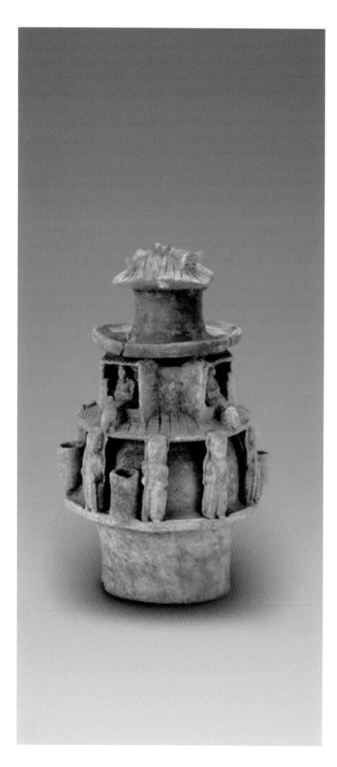

灰陶魂瓶

西晋

泥质灰陶质

腹径 21.6 厘米，通高 34 厘米

Grey Pottery Soul Bottle

Western Jin Dynasty

Grey Pottery

Belly Diameter 21.6 cm/ Height 34 cm

魂瓶为泥质灰陶冥器，整体由四层构成，顶层与瓶身分制，作四阿式顶，圆形屋，下承圆盘；第二层为四面塑一层龛，龛内各塑一坐像，旁立一侍童，龛前各立一鸟，昂首对立，生动有趣；第三层正面开门，门两侧设叠檐歇山顶双高阙，四周分塑4个圆筒状小罐，其间塑6身立像；底层为束腰圆座。此魂瓶的西晋墓中，有"元康七年七月十日""广陵郡舆县张平"铭文砖。1981年仪征胥浦93号汉墓出土。

扬州博物馆藏

The soul bottle, made from clay, is a funerary grey pottery object. It has four layers. The round rooftop is separated from its body with a round plate beneath. On the second layer are four shrines in four directions, in which there is a sitting statue respectively with a page boy standing by. Meanwhile a bird is standing in front of each shrine, facing to its master, which makes the composition of art vivid and interesting. There are four small cylindrical jars and six statues standing on the third layer. The bottom layer is a round base with slender waist. The tomb of Western Jin dynasty, from which the soul bottle was unearthed, has a stone tablet with epigraph written "Yuan Kang Qi Nian Qi Yue Shi Ri" and "Guang Ling Zhen Yu Xian Zhang Ping". The bottle was excavated from No. 93 tomb of Han Dynasty at Xupu in Yizheng.

Preserved in Yangzhou Museum

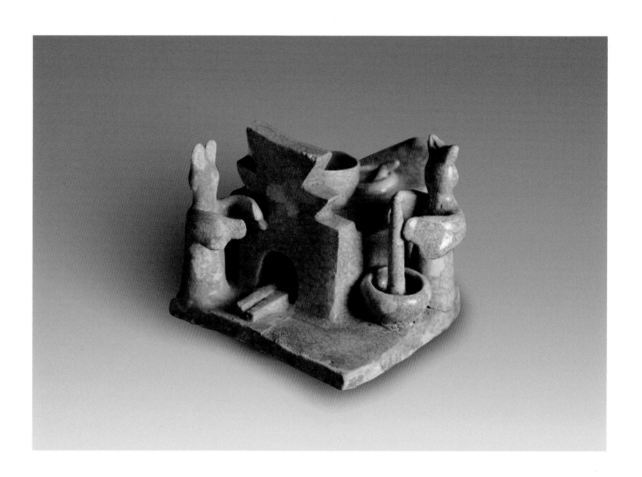

青瓷饮灶模型

西晋

青瓷质

底长 19 厘米，宽 12 厘米，高 14 厘米

Celadon Cooking Stove Model

Western Jin Dynasty

Celadon

Bottom Length 19 cm/ Width 12 cm/ Heigh 14 cm

灶台上塑有大小炊具各一，台前高筑凸形灶壁，壁下中部有倒 U 字形灶口，口内有两块柴火。灶台左侧塑一高髻长裙女子，双臂环抱似填柴状。灶台右侧放置乳钵一个，一高髻女子双手执杵作捣物状。此模型生动地表现了捣药、煎煮药等制药过程。

北京御生堂中医药博物馆藏

The stove is coated with different sizes of cookers and the convex stove wall with U-shaped stove mouth built in the front of stove. The stove mouth the middle of wall contains two pieces of firewood. A woman with high bun and long dress stood on the left of stove and took the pestle for smashing medicine. The encircled arms seem to stuff the firewood. A mortar is set on the right of the stove. This model vividly shows the process of smashing and boiling medicine.

Preserved in Chinese Medicine Museum of Beijing Yu Sheng Tang Drugstore

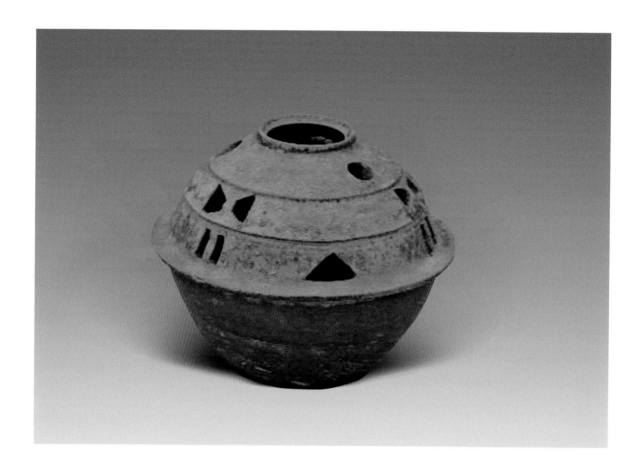

青瓷香熏

西晋

瓷质

直径 16 厘米，高 16 厘米

Celadon Burner of Aromatherapy

Western Jin Dynasty

Porcelain

Diameter 16 cm/ Height 16 cm

子母口，钵形器身，盖宽折沿，盖顶处有大圆孔一个，其周有两弦纹，将盖身均分三份，从上至下依次有小圆孔、成对梯形孔、三角形孔和长方形孔间刻其中。古人熏制天然香草料，用于疾病预防和居室卫生，是现在"治未病"思想和"预防医学"的见证物。

北京御生堂中医药博物馆藏

The burner has a cluster mouth, a bowl-shaped body and a widely folded rim. At the top of the lid, there is a round hole which is carved with two raised ring dividing the body into three segments. From the top to the bottom, there were small holes, double ladder-shaped holes, triangle hole and rectangle hole in the middle. It was used for smoking the natural spice, which can prevent disease and enhance indoor sanitation. It was the witness of the idea of "Disease Prevention" and "Preventive Medicine".

Preserved in Chinese Medicine Museum of Beijing Yu Sheng Tang Drugstore

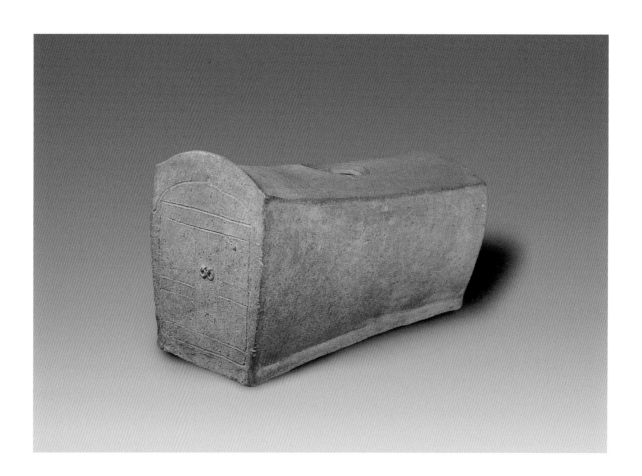

青瓷骨灰罐

晋

瓷质

长 38 厘米，前宽 18.5 厘米，前高 22.5 厘米，后宽 16.5 厘米，后高 17 厘米

Celadon Urn

Jin Dynasty

Porcelain

Length 38 cm/ Front Width 18.5 cm/ Front Height 22.5 cm/ Back Width 16.5 cm/ Back Height 17 cm

前宽后窄，形似棺。前部饰有双开门户，上有
凸出门环。器顶有圆孔，为装骨灰之口，原有
盖已失。浙江省绍兴出土。

上海中医药博物馆藏

This urn is in the shape of a coffin with wide
front and narrow rear. The front part of the
urn is decorated with a double door unit,
fastened by a protruding door knocker. On
the top is a circular hole for containing bone
ash. The original cover of this urn is lost. It
was excavated from Shaoxing City, Zhejiang
Province.

Preserved in Shanghai Museum of Traditional
Chinese Medicine

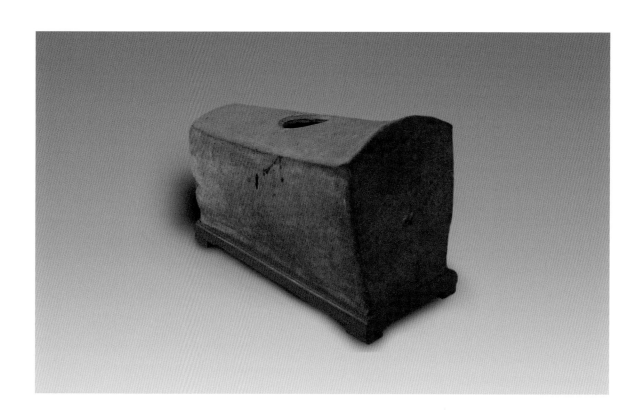

櫬椟

晋

陶质

大头：长 37.6 厘米，宽 23.2 厘米，高 18.3 厘米

小头：长 37.6 厘米，宽 17.8 厘米，高 16.1 厘米

Cinerary Casket

Jin Dynasty

Pottery

Front: Length 37.6 cm/ Width 23.2 cm/ Height 18.3 cm

Back: Length 37.6 cm/ Width 17.8 cm/ Height 16.1 cm

该藏灰陶制成，呈棺形，上部留一孔用于盛装死
者骨灰，大头侧面浅刻门状图案，工艺一般。盛
装骨灰的容器。1955 年入藏。保存基本完好。

中华医学会 / 上海中医药大学医史博物馆藏

This coffin-shaped casket made from grey
pottery has a hole on the top, which is designed
to contain bone ash. The front side is incised
with the motif of a door by shallow carving in
ordinary workmanship. The coffin-shaped casket
is designed for holding bone ash. It was collected
in 1955 and is still in good shape.

Preserved in Chinese Medical Association/Museum
of Chinese Medicine, Shanghai University of
Traditional Chinese Medicine

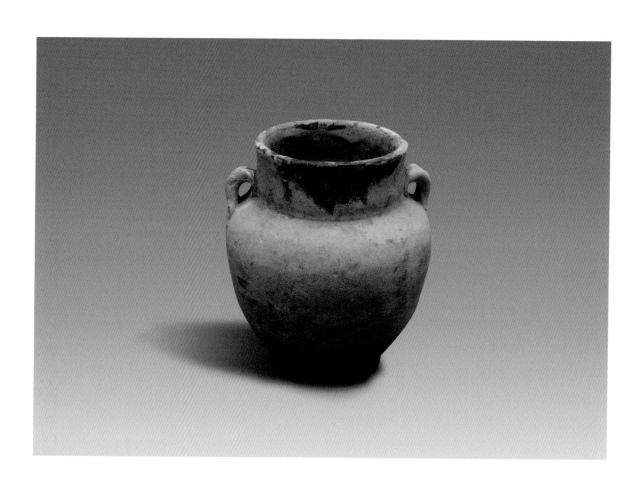

双耳罐

南北朝

陶质

口径 6 厘米，高 96 厘米

Double-Eared Jar

Northern and Southern Dynasties

Pottery

Mouth Diameter 6 cm/ Height 96 cm

圆口，直颈，鼓肩，腹稍内收，平底，有双桥
形耳。由四川省文管所调拨。

成都中医药大学中医药传统文化博物馆藏

The jar has a circular mouth, a straight neck,
a drum-shaped shoulder, a gradually tapering
belly, a flat bottom and double bridge-shaped
ears. The jar was allocated from Sichuan
Administration Committee of Cultural Relics.

Preserved in Museum of Traditional Chinese
Medicine Culture, Chengdu University of Traditional
Chinese Medicine

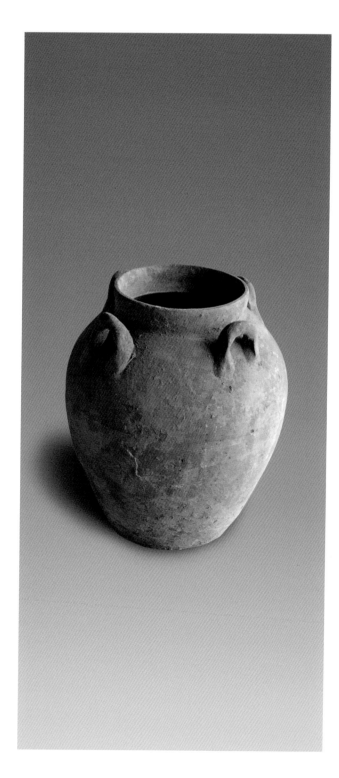

四系罐

南北朝

陶质

口径 10 厘米，底径 10.5 厘米，高 20 厘米

Jar with Four Rings

Northern and Southern Dynasties

Pottery

Mouth Diameter 10 cm/ Bottom Diameter 10.5 cm/

Height 20 cm

直口，鼓肩，腹稍内收，平底，肩部有四个桥
形系。上半部施釉。由成都市考古队调拨。

　　成都中医药大学中医药传统文化博物馆藏

This jar has a straight mouth, a drum-shaped
shoulder, a slightly tapered abdomen and a flat
bottom. Four bridge-shaped rings are attached
to the shoulder and the upper part of the jar is
glazed. The jar was allocated from the Chengdu
Municipal Archaeological Team.

Preserved in Museum of Traditional Chinese
Medicine Culture, Chengdu University of Traditional
Chinese Medicine

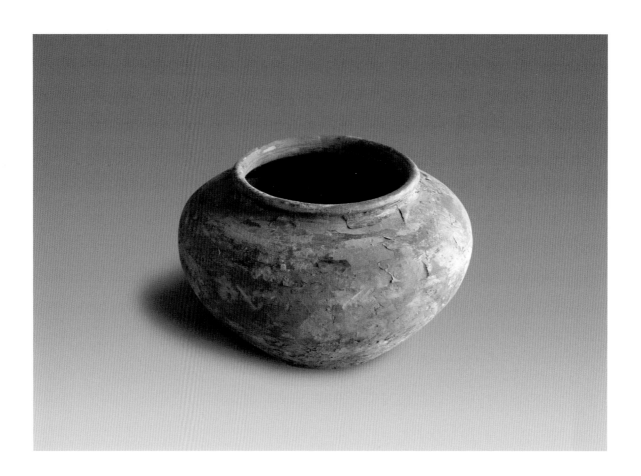

罐

南北朝

陶质

口径 13 厘米，底径 11 厘米，高 14 厘米

Jar

Northern and Southern Dynasties

Pottery

Mouth Diameter 13 cm/ Bottom Diameter 11 cm/ Height 14 cm

圆口，鼓腹，下部内收，平底。上半部施黄釉，由成都市考古队调拨。

成都中医药大学中医药传统文化博物馆藏

This jar is characterized by a circular mouth, a drum abdomen with its lower part narrowing down, a flat bottom, and a yellow-glazed upper part. It was allocated from the Chengdu Municipal Archaeological Team.

Preserved in Museum of Traditional Chinese Medicine Culture, Chengdu University of Traditional Chinese Medicine

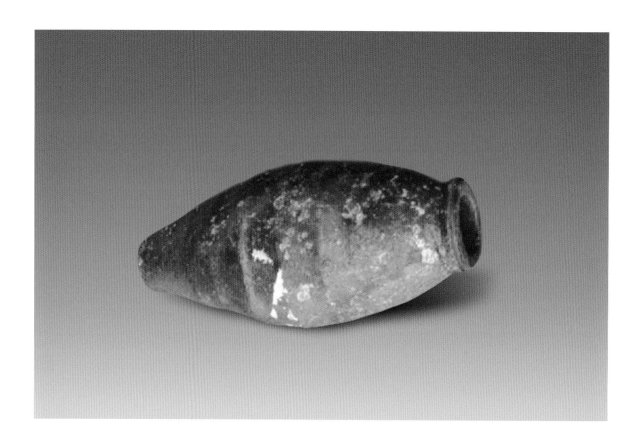

军持

南北朝

陶质

外口径 3.3 厘米，腹径 9.2 厘米，底径 3.5 厘米，通高 20 厘米，壶深 18 厘米，重 362.5 克

Knudika

Northern and Southern Dynasties

Pottery

Outer Mouth Diameter 3.3 cm/ Belly Diameter 9.2 cm/ Bottom Diameter 3.5 cm/ Height 20 cm/ Depth 18 cm/
Weight 362.5 g

平口，鼓腹，腹深，腹下部内敛，平底。军持一词来源于印度梵语，佛教僧侣饮水、洗手等的容器。此物原题"军持"待考。

广东中医药博物馆藏

This knudika has a flat mouth, a deep drum abdomen with its lower part slightly convergent inward, and a flat bottom. The word "knudika" originated from the Indian Sanskrit, meaning a kind of water container used by Buddhist monks for drinking and washing hands. The original name of this object remains to be verified.

Preserved in Guangdong Chinese Medicine Museum

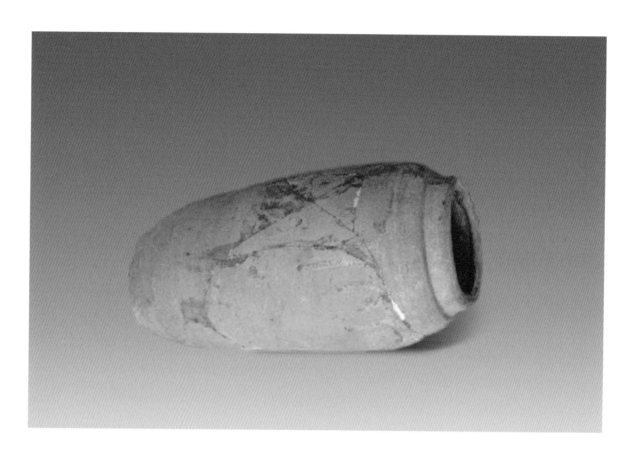

军持

南北朝

陶质

外口径 6.3 厘米，腹径 11.5 厘米，底径 7.5 厘米，通高 22.23 厘米，壶深 22 厘米，重 880 克

Knudika

Northern and Southern Dynasties

Pottery

Outer Mouth Diameter 6.3 cm/ Belly Diameter 11.5 cm/ Bottom Diameter 7.5 cm/ Height 22.23 cm/ Depth 22 cm/ Weight 880 g

平口，鼓腹，腹深，腹下部内敛，平底。"军持"
一词来源于印度梵语，佛教僧侣饮水、洗手等
的容器。此物原题"军持"待考。

广东中医药博物馆藏

This knudika has a flat mouth, a deep drum
abdomen with its lower part slightly convergent
inward, and a flat bottom. The word "knudika"
originated from the Indian Sanskrit, meaning
the vessel held by Buddhist monks for drinking
and washing hands. The original name of this
object remains to be verified.

Preserved in Guangdong Chinese Medicine Museum

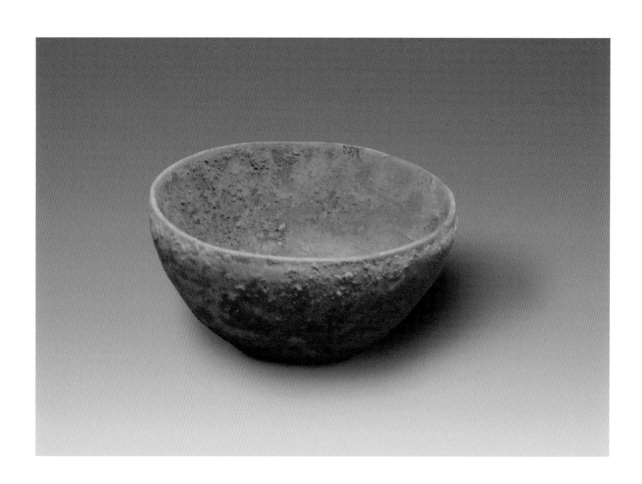

杯

南北朝

瓷质

径 9 厘米，高 5 厘米

Cup

Northern and Southern Dynasties

Porcelain

Diameter 9 cm/ Height 5 cm

圆口，直腹，平底，施青釉。饮酒用具。由万州区文物管理所调拨。

成都中医药大学中医药传统文化博物馆藏

This green-glazed cup, with a round mouth, a straight belly and a flat bottom, was used as a wine container. It was allocated from Wanzhou District Administration Committee of Cultural Relics.

Preserved in Museum of Traditional Chinese Medicine Culture, Chengdu University of Traditional Chinese Medicine

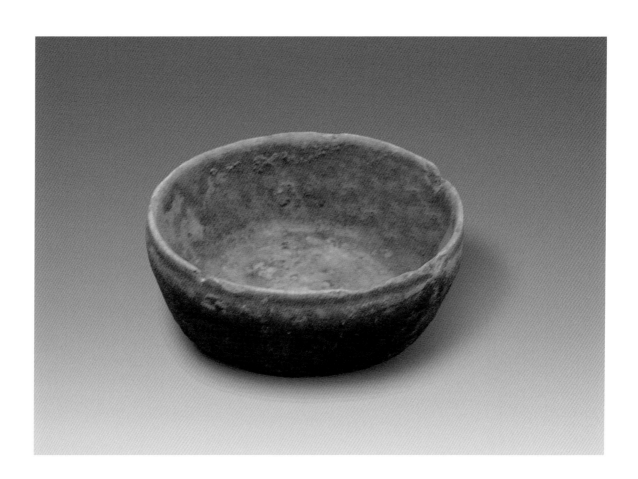

杯

南北朝

瓷质

径 9 厘米，高 5 厘米

Cup

Northern and Southern Dynasties

Porcelain

Diameter 9 cm/ Height 5 cm

圆口直腹，平底，施青釉。饮酒用具。由万州区文物管理所调拨。

　　成都中医药大学中医药传统文化博物馆藏

This green-glazed cup with a round mouth, a straight belly and a flat bottom, was used as a wine container. It was allocated from Wanzhou District Administration Committee of Cultural Relics.

Preserved in Museum of Traditional Chinese Medicine Culture, Chengdu University of Traditional Chinese Medicine

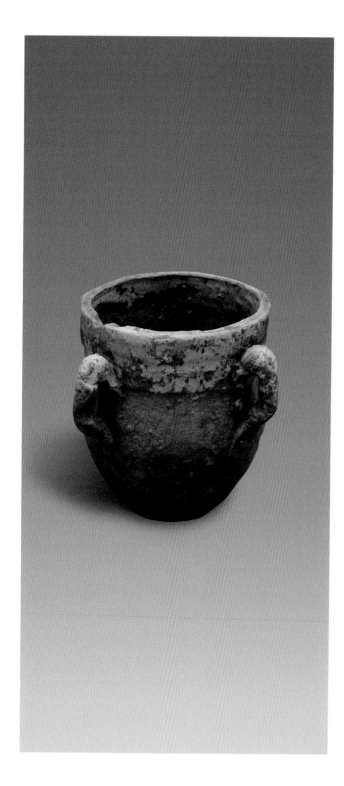

四耳罐

南北朝

陶质

腹径 9.5 厘米，高 22 厘米

Jar with Four Ears

Northern and Southern Dynasties

Pottery

Belly Diameter 9.5 cm/ Height 22 cm

直腹，平底，均匀分布四个桥形耳。由四川省

文管会调拨。

　　成都中医药大学中医药传统文化博物馆藏

This jar has a straight belly and a flat bottom.
Four bridge-shaped handles are distributed
evenly around the body. The jar was allocated
from Sichuan Administration Committee of
Cultural Relics.

Preserved in Museum of Traditional Chinese
Medicine Culture, Chengdu University of Traditional
Chinese Medicine

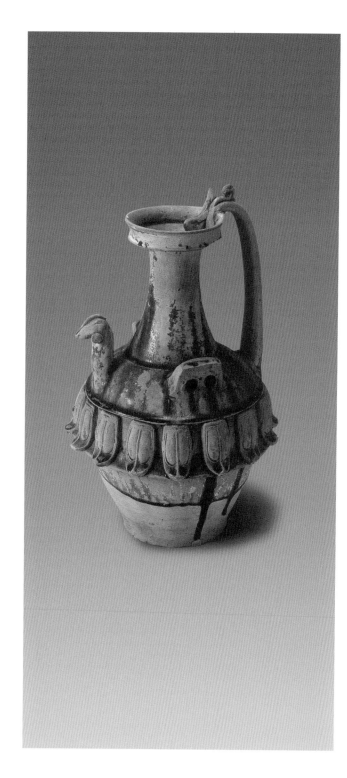

青釉覆莲鸡首壶

南朝

瓷质

口径 11.2 厘米，高 23 厘米

Celadon Ewer with Chicken-head Spout and Downward Facing Lotus

Southern Dynasty

Porcelain

Mouth Diameter 11.2 cm/ Height 23 cm

小盘口，细颈，扁球腹。肩部饰凸起弦纹。腹部贴饰一周覆莲瓣纹。前置鸡首，鸡突目，尖嘴，长颈，后置圆形鋬，两侧置双孔桥形横系。半施青釉，底部无釉，有流釉现象。1972 年扬州市西湖荷叶王庄出土。

扬州博物馆藏

With embossed string patterns decorating the shoulder, the ewer has a small plate-shaped mouth, a thin neck, and an oblate spheroid abdomen embellished with scrolling downward-facing lotus petals in relief. The spout, opposite to a circular handle, is in the shape of a chicken head with protruding eyes, a pointed beak and a long neck. Horizontal ears in the shape of a double-arch bridge are placed at both sides. Sagging glaze appears on the upper half of the celadon-glazed ewer. The bottom is unglazed. The ewer was unearthed from Wangzhuang Manor at Lotus Leaf Village at West Lake County in Yangzhou City, Jiangsu Province. Preserved in Yangzhou Museum

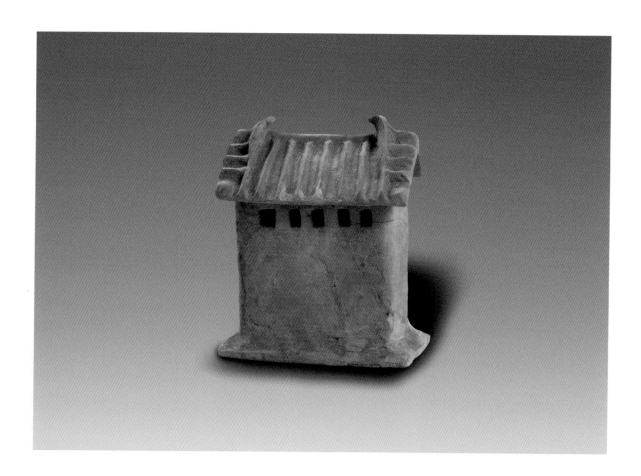

陶屋

南朝

陶质

长 17.5 厘米，宽 10.7 厘米，高 20.5 厘米

Pottery House

Southern Dynasty

Porcelain

Length 17.5 cm/ Width 10.7 cm/ Height 20.5 cm

长方形，两坡顶，屋脊有升起曲线，并饰鸱尾。顶梁挑角内弯。在陶屋一面近屋檐部并列五个方形小窗。平底，宽出屋身。在六朝墓葬中随葬大量生活明器，这陶屋就是当时人"事死如事生"的实物明证。南京郊区出土。

南京博物院藏

This rectangular pottery house has a double pitch roof with upturned roof ridge in the shape of owl tails. The introverting roof beam is in pick angle. There are five square windows on the upper part of the pottery house near the eaves. The bottom of the house is flat and wider than the main part. This pottery house was excavated together with many burial objects for daily use, a clear proof of the fact that the people in the Six Dynasties served the dead as they would have served them alive. It was excavated from the suburbs of Nanjing, Jiangsu Province.

Preserved in Nanjing Museum

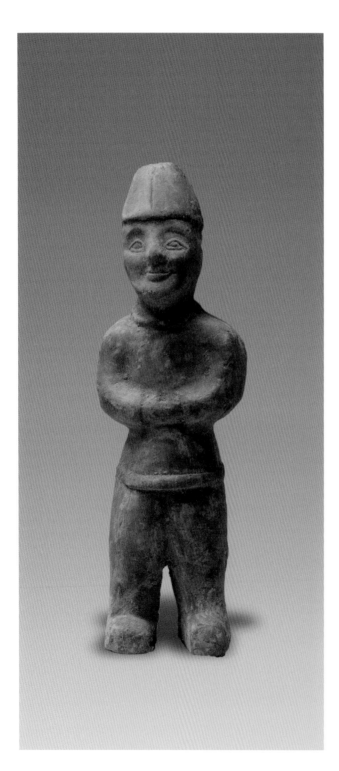

陶男侍俑

南朝

灰陶质

高 21.5 厘米

Pottery Figurine of a Male Servant

Southern Dynasty

Gray Pottery

Height 21.5 cm

侍者造型，上身穿袴褶，头戴近平尖顶有毡帽，张目抿口，抄手直立，面部略带微笑，反映了六朝时代建康城侍役人员的形象特征。南京郊区出土。

南京市夫子庙展览馆藏

The servant with a flat-topped felt cap stands uprightly. He wears a hakama with his hands held in front. He is smiling happily with his eyes open and his mouth closed. It reflects the characteristics of male servants in Jiankang in Southern Dynasty. The figurine was excavated in the suburbs of Nanjing.

Preserved in the Exhibition Hall of Confucius Temple in Nanjing

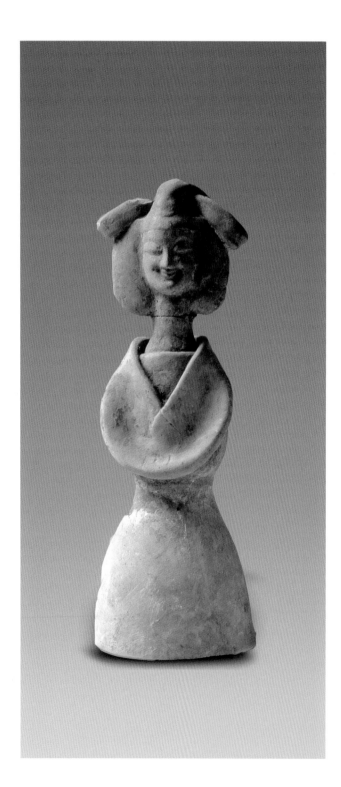

陶女俑

南朝

陶质

高 30.5 厘米

Pottery Figurine of a Woman

Southern Dynasty

Height 30.5 cm

面相丰满，双眼微笑，头上发髻呈长条状向左右伸出，两侧下垂盖压双耳，身着衽衫，内有中衣，窄袖，束腰曳地长裙，双手拱手于腹前。

南京市博物馆藏

The plump smiling woman's hair style is quite special. The upper part of her hair is coiled with two strands of hair extending to the left and the right respectively; while the lower part of her hair droops over her ears. She wears a coat in style of lapel with narrow sleeves and a long skirt with a tight waist. She also wears underlinen within the coat. She holds her two hands in front of the belly.

Preserved in Nanjing Municipal Museum

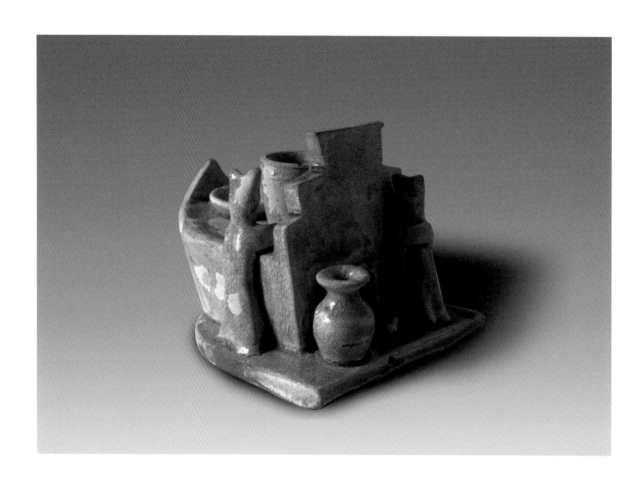

南朝青釉灶具

南朝

瓷质

底长 10.5 厘米，底宽 12 厘米，高 10 厘米

Celadon Cooking Utensils

Southern Dynasty

Porcelain

Bottom Length 10.5 cm/ Bottom Width 12 cm/ Height 10 cm

灶为半断船形，灶面设置炊具三个，前一个直壁深腹，后一个撇口扁腹，另一个设在灶面左侧，为小口半圆腹。灶右侧靠灶旁立一人，双手伸向前，似捧炊具之状。灶前右侧置一瓶，左侧一人拱手而立，是看管灶火之人，灶口置木柴两根，满施青釉，釉闪微黄开小纹片，釉光亮透润，底平无釉，胎浅灰色，胎坚硬。这件明器反映当时社会的生活写照。

陈炎藏

The stove is in the shape of a half boat, on the top of which are three cookers. The one at the front has a straight wall and swollen abdomen, while the rear contains a flared mouth and a flat belly. The cooker on the left side has a small mouth and a semi-circular stomach. To the right side of the stove stands a man, his hands stretching forward, as if holding a cooker. In front of the stove to the right is a bottle, and to the left stands a man with one hand cupped in the other. He seems to be watching over the fire. Two pieces of firewood are put at the stove mouth, to which lustering yellowish crackle glaze is fully applied. The bottom is flat and unglazed. The body is hard and in pale grey. This funerary object is a vivid portrayal of the social life in the Southern Dynasty.

Collected by Chen Yan

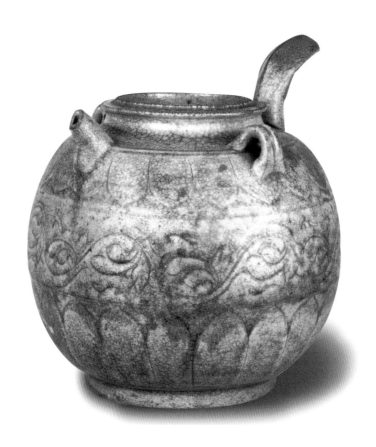

青釉划花单柄壶

南朝

瓷质

口径 11 厘米，底径 12.4 厘米，高 21.3 厘米

Single-handled Celadon Pot with Incised Floral Patterns

Southern Dynasty

Porcelain

Mouth Diameter 11 cm/ Bottom Diameter 12.4 cm/ Height 21.3 cm

壶口折边，短颈，圆腹，平底，肩部两面起双系，有短流，与流相对处置单柄，柄尖高起。肩部及腹下刻画仰覆莲瓣纹各一周，中间卷枝纹，纹饰之间以弦纹隔开。里、外满施青绿色釉，釉厚处透明如玻璃。

故宫博物院藏

The pot has an everted angular rim, a short neck, a swollen abdomen and a flat bottom. Double-loop ears are attached to both sides of the shoulder. With the end raised up, a handle, opposite to the short spout, is placed on the shoulder of the pot. Scrolls of lotus petals are incised beneath both the shoulder and the abdomen with entwining branches in the middle, spaced out by string patterns. The interior and exterior of the pot are fully coated with thick greenish glaze, as transparent as glass.

Preserved in the Palace Museum

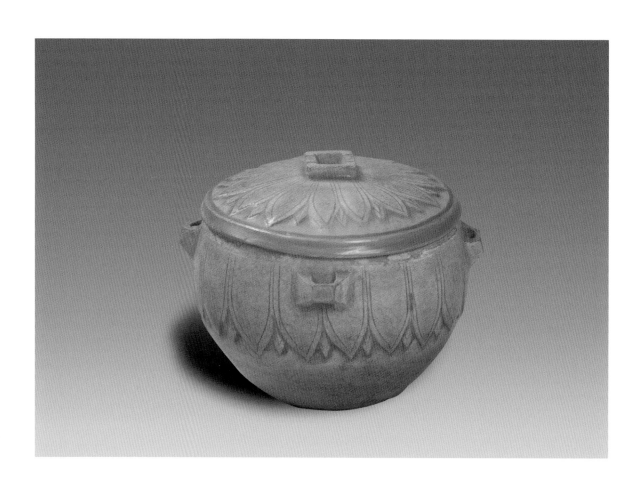

青釉莲瓣纹瓷盖罐

南朝

瓷质

口径 7.3 厘米，底径 3.9 厘米，通高 6.9 厘米

Lidded Celedon Jar with Lotus Patterns

Southern Dynasty

Porcelain

Mouth Diameter 7.3 cm/ Bottom Diameter 3.9 cm/ Height 6.9 cm

胎黄白色，黄绿色釉，罐口稍敛，尖唇，圆球腹，底平略凹，底无釉。有弧形盖，内置子母口，盖顶置四方形钮，并以钮为中心印莲瓣纹一周。罐上腹部有四桥形系，两两对称排列，腹部饰覆莲纹一周，莲瓣瘦长。南京象山二号墓出土。

南京博物院藏

The yellowish white body of the jar is coated with celadon glaze. The jar has a slightly contracted mouth, a tipped lip, a globular belly, and an unglazed bottom which is slightly concave inward. It is covered with a curved snap lid. On the top of the lid is placed a square knob, around which are scroll lotus petals. Based on the symmetrical arrangement, four bridge-shaped handles are placed opposite to each other on the upper abdomen, around which are slim lotus petals in relief. It was excavated from No. 2 Tomb on Mount Xiangshan in Nanjing, Jiangsu Province.

Preserved in Nanjing Museum

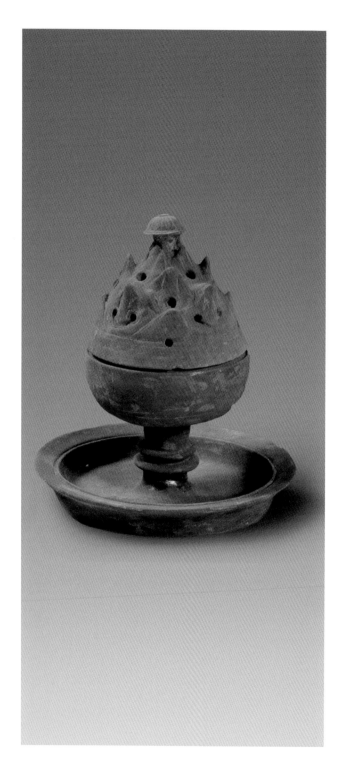

博山式陶香熏

南朝

陶质

口径 10 厘米，底径 9.5 厘米，高 20.5 厘米

Boshan Pottery Censer

Southern Dynasty

Pottery

Mouth Diameter 10 cm/ Bottom Diameter 9.5 cm/

Height 20.5 cm

下部为宽折沿，平底的圆盘。盘中有圆柱形灯柱，柱上有弯曲的把手，把手末端呈侧垂的三角形，灯柱上为圆形、一面敞开的灯盏托，内有釉瓷灯盏。其上有一圆形灯罩，灯罩一面敞开，一面有格窗，灯罩可以转动以便调整照射方向。此陶灯结构合理，造型优美，堪称六朝灯具精品。南京栖霞区前新塘出土。

南京博物院藏

The lower part of this lamp is a plate with a broad outwardly folded edge and a flat bottom. There is a cylinder-shaped lamppost with a curved handle attached to it, ending in a downward triangle leaning to one side. A round lamp holder with one side open is on the top of the post, inside which is a glazed porcelain lamp. A round lampshade with lattice windows on one side and a wide opening on the other can be rotated to provide an adjustable angle of illumination. Reasonably structured and appealing to the eye, this lamp can be rated as a showpiece of the lamps made in the Six Dynasties. It was excavated from Qian Xintang Village in Qixia District of Nanjing. Preserved in Nanjing Museum

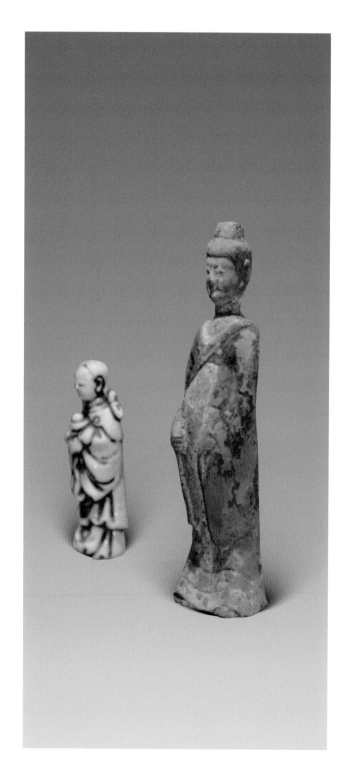

怀孕妇女模型

北魏

瓷质

高 30 厘米

Figurine of Pregnant Woman

Northern Wei Dynasty

Porcelain

Height 30 cm

直立孕妇模型，束髻，面容慈祥，身着右衽衣裙，双手捧腹，体态丰腴，是当时大夫的诊病模型，当时大夫出外给人诊病，尤其是到大户人家给妇人看病，由于男女授受不亲的观念，要由妇人指认不舒服的地方，大夫据此做出判断。

北京御生堂中医药博物馆藏

The standing pregnant female figurine with knotted hair wears a long dress. She looks kind and peaceful. She puts her hands on her round belly. It is the model of diagnosing the disease. At that time, the doctors visited patients and understood their condition based on the part on the figurine pointed by female patients. This was influenced by the traditional virtue value for women especially those in rich families that they should avoid any physical contact with any men except for their father and husband , known as in Chinese "Nan nv shou shou bu qin".

Preserved in Chinese Medicine Museum of Beijing Yu Sheng Tang Drugstore

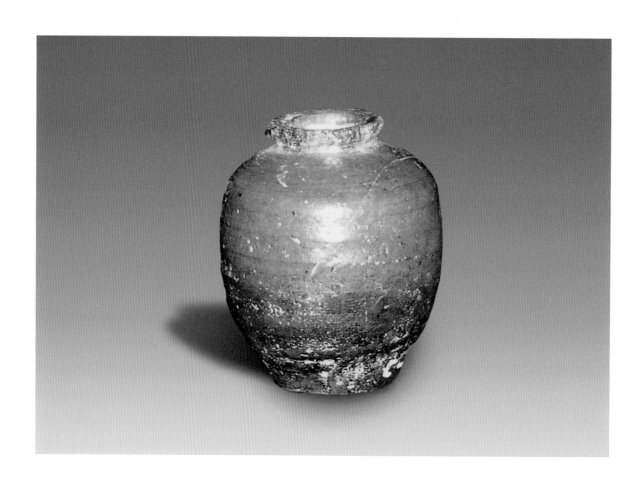

小药瓶

北朝

陶质

口径 2 厘米，底径 2.3 厘米，通高 4.8 厘米，重 50 克

Drug Container

Northern Dynasty

Pottery

Mouth Diameter 2 cm/ Bottom Diameter 2.3 cm/ Height 4.8 cm/ Weight 50 g

小口圆唇，折肩，直腹，拱壁底上三分之二处
有灰釉。药具。完整无损。陕西省鄠邑区征集。

陕西医史博物馆藏

This small-mouthed bottle has a round rim, an
angular shoulder and a straight belly. Two-thirds
above the bottom of the buttress is coated with
ash glaze. The container remains intact. It was
collected from Huyi District, Shaanxi Province.
Preserved in Shaanxi Museum of Medical History

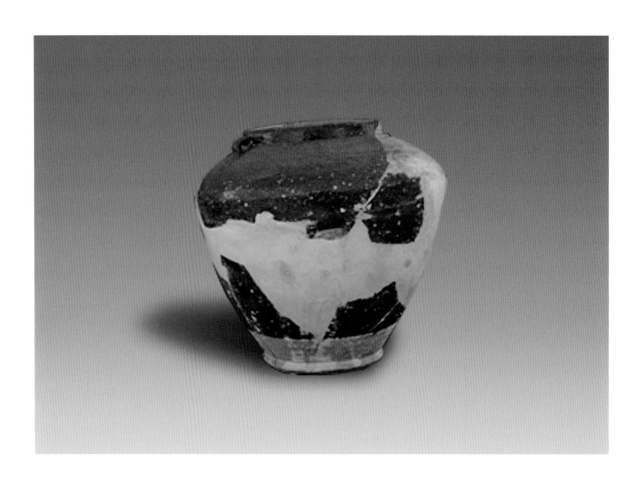

双耳罐

北朝

陶质

口径 15.8 厘米，底径 13.5 厘米，通高 29 厘米，重 4700 克

Double-Eared Jar

Northern Dynasty

Pottery

Mouth Diameter 15.8 cm/ Bottom Diameter 13.5 cm/ Height 29 cm/ Weight 4,700 g

直口，折肩，斜腹，圈足，肩有双耳。盛贮器。有修补。陕西省耀州区孙家垣征集。

陕西医史博物馆藏

The jar has a straight mouth, an angular shoulder, an oblique abdomen, a ring foot, and two ears attached to the shoulder. The jar, used as a container, was restored. It was collected from Sunjiayuan Township at Yaozhou District, Shaanxi Province.

Preserved in Shaanxi Museum of Medical History

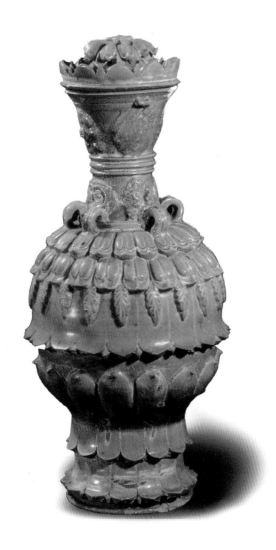

青釉仰覆莲花尊

北朝

瓷质

口径 15.1 厘米，底径 18 厘米，高 54.4 厘米

Celadon Zun Vessel with Lotus-Petal Design

Northern Dynasty

Porcelain

Mouth Diameter 15.1 cm/ Bottom Diameter

18 cm/ Height 54.4 cm

胎灰白细密，施化妆土，釉色青中闪绿。喇叭口，长束颈，椭圆形腹，圈足，莲花状盖。颈部饰三道凸弦纹和六个贴花团龙，颈，肩处有六个双环形系，肩部堆塑两周双瓣覆莲，腹部饰垂叶纹及仰覆莲各一周，足部为两周覆莲。莲瓣均丰满肥硕，向外微卷，造型端庄，装饰富丽，是北朝青瓷中典型的器物。

河北博物院藏

The greyish white body of the Zun vessel is of fine texture. Painted with engobe, the vessel is glazed turquoise. It has a trumpet mouth, a long contracted neck, an oval belly, a ring foot and a lotus-shaped lid. The neck is decorated with three convexing string motifs and six applique dragons. Between the neck and shoulder are six crossed circular rings. Two bands of downward scrolling lotus with dual petals are pasted around the shoulder, with a band of upward lotus together with drooping leaf pattern around the belly, and two more bands of downward lotus are placed around the foot. All the lotus petals are chubby and fleshy, slightly curving outward. With both the demure design and splendid decoration, this celadon Zun vessel is typical of celadon ware in the Northern Dynasty.

Preserved in Hebei Museum

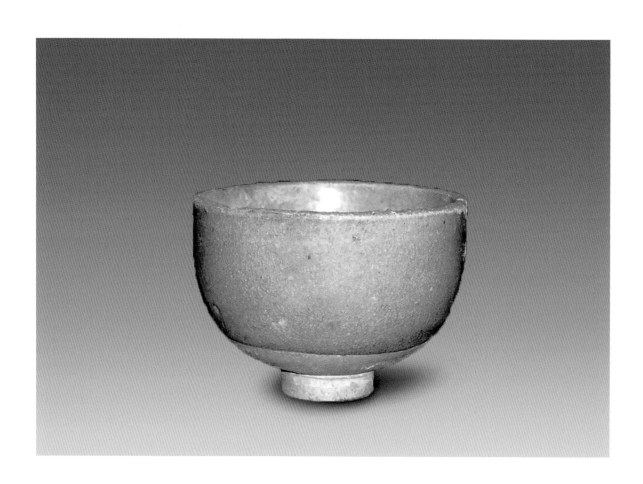

青釉瓷碗

北朝

青釉瓷质

口径 8.7 厘米，底径 3 厘米，通高 6.4 厘米，重 200 克

Celadon Bowl

Northern Dynasty

Porcelain

Mouth Diameter 8.7 cm/ Bottom Diameter 3 cm/ Height 6.4 cm/ Weight 200 g

直口，直腹，小平底，黄釉，底部无釉。食具，
生活用器具。三级文物，有裂口。1987 年入藏。
陕西省澄城县善化乡征集。

陕西医史博物馆藏

This yellow-glazed bowl has a straight mouth, a
straight belly and an unglazed tiny flat bottom.
Used as tableware and household ware, the
celadon bowl with a cleft is classified as third-
class cultural relics. It was collected from
Chengcheng County, Shaanxi Province, in
1987.

Preserved in Shaanxi Museum of Medical History

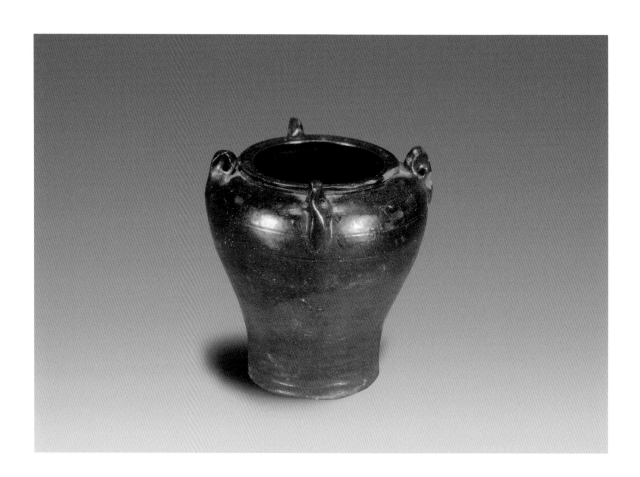

黑褐釉四系罐

北齐

瓷质

口径 9.4 厘米，底径 8 厘米，高 14 厘米

Blackish-brown-glazed Jar with Four Rings

Northern Qi Dynasty

Porcelain

Mouth Diameter 9.4 cm/ Bottom Diameter 8 cm/ Height 14 cm

胎质坚硬，呈砖红色。满施黑褐釉，上浓下淡，釉面莹润光亮。敛口，广肩深腹，下腹内收至底渐宽，平底。肩部有四系，均高出口沿，上腹部有两周浅弦纹。

河北博物院藏

The brick-red body is hard and is fully coated with bright and smooth blackish brown glaze, with the colour toned down from top to bottom. The jar is designed with a contracted mouth, a broad shoulder and a deep belly which gradually narrows down but extends slightly at the bottom. There are four loop handles on the shoulder, slightly higher than the mouth rim. The upper abdomen of the jar is decorated with two bands of shallow string patterns.

Preserved in Hebei Museum

◈ 第二章　隋　唐

Chapter Two　Sui and Tang Dynasties

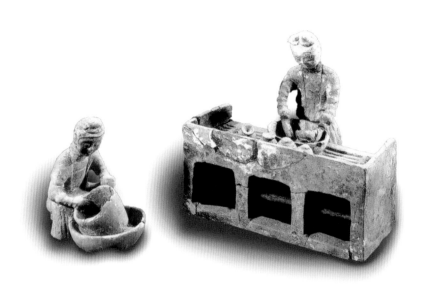

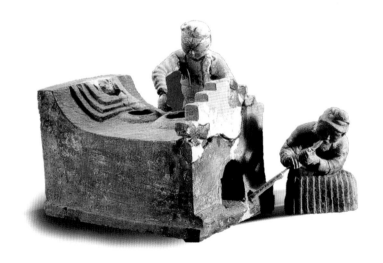

灰陶炊事俑

隋

陶质

厨俑：高 14 厘米

灶：长 22 厘米，宽 10.2 厘米，高 14.3 厘米

洗涤台：长 23 厘米，宽 10.2 厘米，高 10.6 厘米

俑皆着紧身衣，一俑头顶盘做单髻，蹲于盆前洗甑；一俑头顶盘做双髻，立于长案大盆前洗碗；一俑立于灶前，做炒菜状；一俑蹲于灶前，双手持一吹火筒吹火。这组炊事俑造型生动，朴实自然，生动地表现出当时人们的饮食生活。湖北武昌出土。

湖北省博物馆藏

Grey Pottery Cooking Figurines

Sui Dynasty

Pottery

Cooking Figurine: Height 14 cm

Cooking Stove: Length 22 cm/ Width 10.2 cm/ Height 14.3 cm

Washing Sink: Length 23 cm/ Width 10.2 cm/ Height 10.6 cm

This set of pottery figurines, simple but vivid, reflect the dietetic life in the Sui dynasty. The four men are all in corsetry. One man with single topknot is squatting in front of a basin, washing rice steamer. Another man with double topknots is standing in front of a large sink, washing bowls. In front of the stove stands a third man, cooking, while beside him is another man holding a blowtube, squatting and blowing the fire. They were excavated from Wuchang city, Hubei province.

Preserved in Hubei Provincial Museum

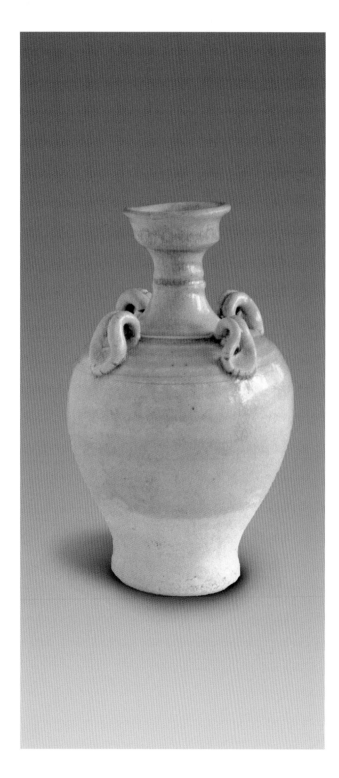

白釉四耳盘口瓶

隋

瓷质

高 20.3 厘米

White-glazed Bottle with Dish-shaped Mouth and Four Ears

Sui Dynasty

Porcelain

Height 20.3 cm

盘口微外侈，细颈，丰肩，平底，肩部饰并条
钮眼形耳四只，颈部饰二周凸弦纹，耳下部饰
三周细弦纹。施白釉至腹下，不到底，有细开片。
灰白胎。各部分比例恰当，造型优美。

关世钊藏

The bottle has a slightly flared dish-shaped mouth, a narrow neck, a flattened shoulder and a flat bottom. Four button-shaped double-cord ears are placed on the shoulder. Its neck is decorated with two convex bowstring patterns and the part beneath the handles displays three thin bowstring patterns. The greyish-white body is white-glazed with small crackles, while the lower part of its belly and the bottom are left unglazed. The bottle looks beautiful and well-proportioned.

Collected by Guan Shizhao

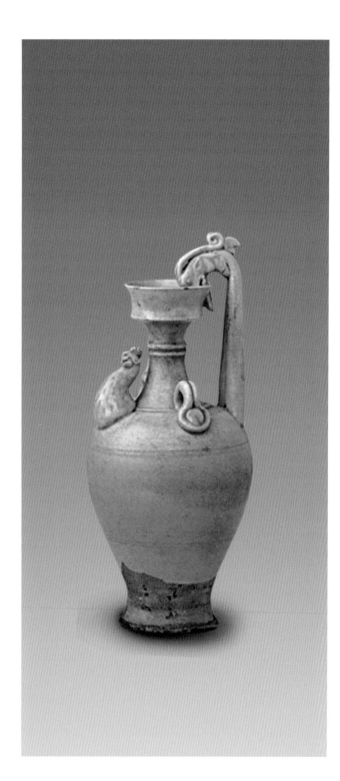

鸡首壶

隋

白瓷质

口径 7.1 厘米，高 27.4 厘米

Chicken-head Ewer

Sui Dynasty

White Porcelain

Mouth Diameter 7.1 cm/ Height 27.4 cm

盘口外侈，圆唇，束腰式细长颈，丰肩，鼓腹下渐收，平底。肩部一侧塑一鸡首，高冠圆目，昂首张口作啼鸣状，与之相对一侧为直体曲颈形龙柄，龙口衔接壶口沿。肩部置对称式环形耳。1957年陕西西安李静训墓出土。

中国国家博物馆藏

The ewer has a dish-shaped mouth with the rim slightly turning outward, a thin and long neck with a contracted waistline, a round shoulder, a drum belly gradually narrowing down and a flat bottom. A round-eyed rooster head with a tall cockscomb is pasted on one side of the shoulder, the chest of which is holding high, like crowing with the open beak. On the other side is a dragon-shaped handle with straight body and bend neck, whose mouth is connected with the ewer's rim. Two ring ears are symmetrically placed on the shoulder of the ewer. The pot was unearthed from the tomb of Li Jingxun, Xi'an, Shaanxi Province, in 1957. Preserved in National Museum of China

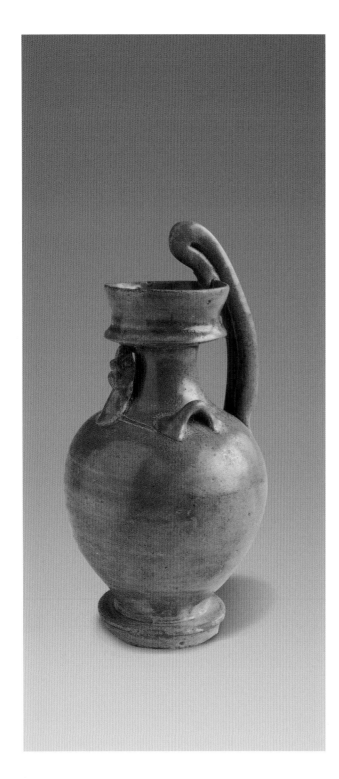

青釉鸡首壶

隋

瓷质

高 18.5 厘米

Celadon Chicken-head Ewer

Sui Dynasty

Porcelain

Height 18.5 cm

冼口，细颈，丰腹，平底。肩部设鸡形为首，后设圆状条为把，高出口缘。两边附对称桥形耳。青釉微闪灰，莹润透亮，胎细坚硬，白中闪灰。

杨振达藏

The ewer is characterized with a basin-shaped mouth, a narrow neck, a bulging belly, and a flat bottom. On the shoulder is a round long handle with its upper end shaped into a chicken head and set just above the mouth rim. The upper part of the vessel is flanked by a pair of bridge-shaped ears. The celadon is bright and lustrous with slight tints of grey. Its white greyish body is of fine and hard texture.

Collected by Yang Zhenda

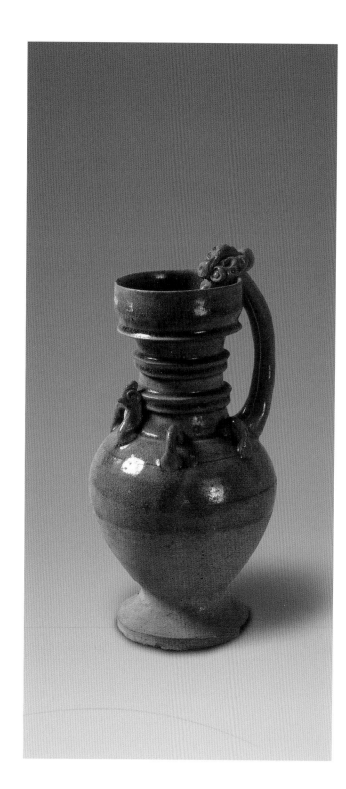

青釉鸡首龙柄壶

隋

瓷质

口径 7 厘米，腹径 11.7 厘米，底径 7.9 厘米，
高 22 厘米

Celadon Chicken-head Ewer with Dragon Handle

Sui Dynasty

Porcelain

Mouth Diameter 7 cm/ Belly Diameter 11.7 cm/

Bottom Diameter 7.9 cm/ Height 22 cm

圆唇，浅盘口，细长颈，颈上箍有三道凸棱。溜肩，长圆腹，胫部收敛，圈足。肩部饰 4 个对称桥耳，一侧塑一鸡首，鸡翘首远望，与鸡首相对为一龙柄，龙眼圆睁，低首张口衔壶，内外均施釉，青翠莹润，釉面光洁，有细小开片，腹部以下无釉，为隋代典型器。1976 年仪征刘集红光村出土。

仪征博物馆藏

The ewer has a round lip, a shallow pot-shaped mouth, and a slender neck, on which are hooped three ridge lines. It is also characterized with a sloping shoulder, a long, round belly, a shin tapering downward and a ring foot. Its shoulder is decorated with two pairs of symmetrical bridge-shaped ears. A raised chicken head is sculpted on one side of the pot, and to its opposite is a handle in the shape of a dragon. The dragon, eyes wide-open and head lowered, opens its mouth to hold the ewer. Its inner and outer surfaces are coated with bright, smooth and verdant glaze with small crackles. The lower part of its belly is unglazed. The ewer is typical of porcelain ware made in the Sui Dynasty, and was unearthed from Hongguang Village, Liuji Township, Yizheng, Jiangsu Province, in the year 1976.
Preserved in Yi Zheng Museum

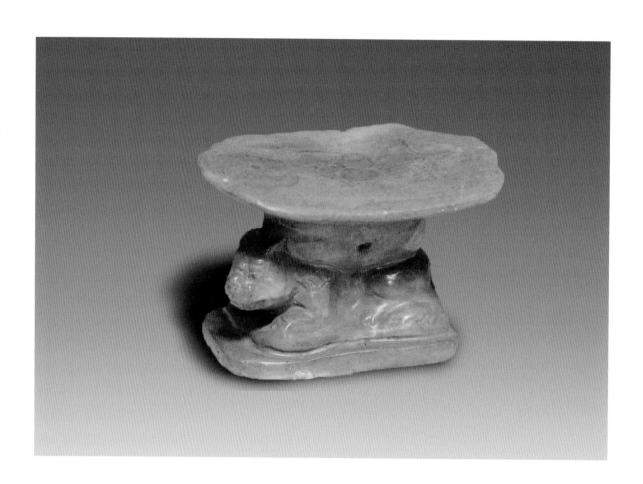

脉枕

唐

瓷质

长 14 厘米，宽 9.5 厘米，高 9 厘米

Wrist Cushion

Tang Dynasty

Porcelain

Length 14 cm/ Width 9.5 cm/ Height 9 cm

枕上层为不规则长圆形，并向一侧稍倾斜之，面上有三朵四瓣花纹。中层为一卧虎。底层为长方形座板。医生为病人切脉用。浙江宁波市和义路出土。

浙江宁波保国寺文管会藏

The upper part of this cushion is in the shape of an irregular ellipse with an inclined lateral side. There are three quatrefoil floral patterns on the upper surface. The middle part of this cushion is shaped into a crouching tiger. The lower part of it is a rectangle-shaped base. This cushion, on which a patient could rest his or her wrist for the doctor to feel the pulse, was excavated from Heyi Road, Ningbo City, Zhejiang Province. Preserved in the Department of Cultural Relics Conservation of Baoguo Temple, Ningbo City, Zhejiang Province

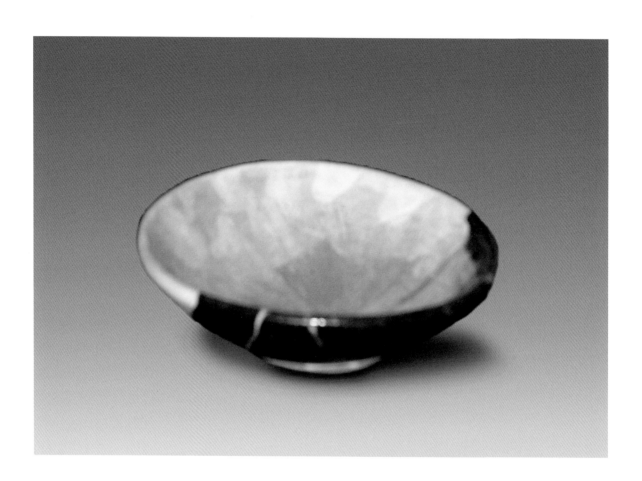

瓷研砵

唐

瓷质

口径 17 厘米，底径 7.5 厘米，通高 5 厘米，重 300 克

Porcelain Mortar

Tang Dynasty

Porcelain

Mouth Diameter 17 cm/ Bottom Diameter 7.5 cm/ Height 5 cm/ Weight 300 g

敛口，斜腹，圈足，黑釉，钵内无釉。研药器具。

有修补。陕西省铜川市征集。

陕西医史博物馆藏

This mortar has a contracted mouth, an oblique abdomen and a ring foot. Its outside is covered with black glaze, but the interior wall is unglazed. The mortar was an implement for pestling medicine into powder. It was restored and collected from Tongchuan City, Shaanxi Province.

Preserved in Shaanxi Museum of Medical History

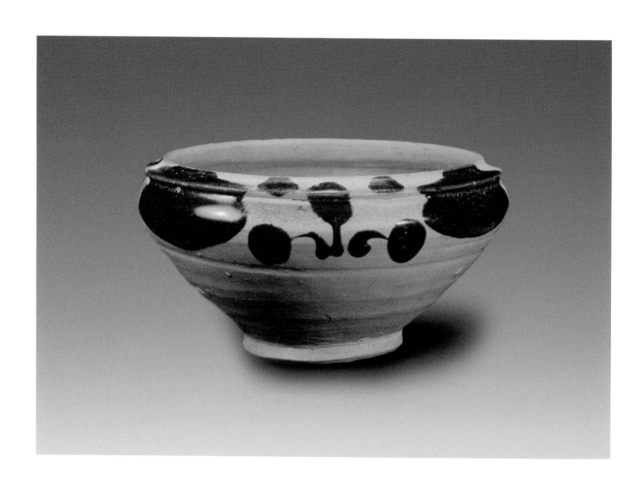

点釉研钵

唐

瓷质

口径 12.7 厘米，腹径 15.1 厘米，足径 6.6 厘米，高 8.12 厘米

Dot-glazed Mortar

Tang Dynasty

Porcelain

Mouth Diameter 12.7 cm/ Belly Diameter 15.1 cm/ Foot Diameter 6.6 cm/ Height 8.12 cm

通体白胎，只在外肩饰黑釉数点，简洁明快。

陕西咸阳出土。

陕西医史博物馆藏

The vessel has an entirely white body with only several black-glazed dots decorating its shoulder in a concise and lively style. It was unearthed in Xianyang, Shaanxi Province.

Preserved in Shaanxi Museum of Medical History

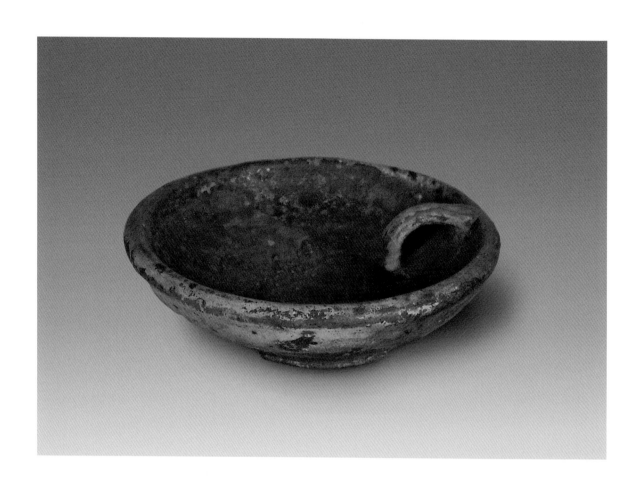

瓷油盏

唐

瓷质

口外径 11.8 厘米，通高 1.35 厘米

Porcelain Oil Lamp

Tang Dynasty

Porcelain

Mouth Outer Diameter 11.8 cm/ Height 1.35 cm

碟形，施黑釉，为唐永和窑制作，工艺粗糙，施釉不匀，底及外侧下半部均无釉，盏内有环状系。盏有使用痕迹，盏底无款识。1964 年入藏。制药工具。保存基本完好。

中华医学会 / 上海中医药大学医史博物馆藏

The oil lamp, in the shape of a small dish, was used as a pharmaceutical tool. Coated with black glaze, it was a production of Yonghe kiln in the Tang Dynasty. Due to coarse craftwork, the glaze was enameled unevenly, and its bottom and the lower part of its outside are left unglazed. Ring-like traces can be found inside it. There are signs showing that it had been used before, and there is no seal on the bottom. Collected in the year 1964, the object has been kept intact.
Preserved in Chinese Medical Association/ Museum of Chinese Medicine, Shanghai University of Traditional Chinese Medicine

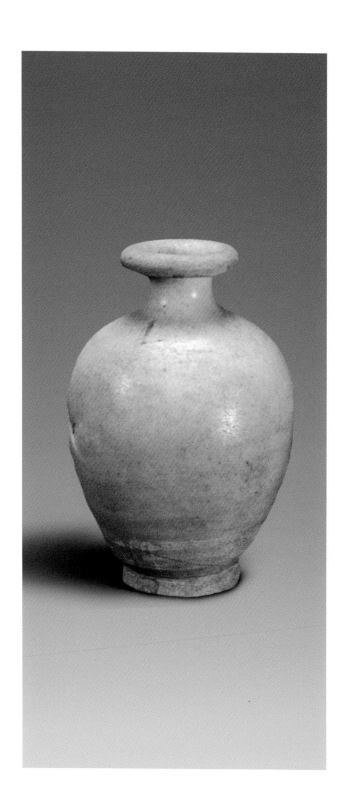

白瓷药瓶

唐

瓷质

口径 2.5 厘米，底径 2.7 厘米，腹围 7 厘米，

通高 7.7 厘米，颈高 2 厘米

White-glazed Medicine Bottle

Tang Dynasty

Porcelain

Mouth Diameter 2.5 cm/ Bottom Diameter

2.7cm/ Belly Girth 7 cm/ Total Height 7.7 cm/

Neck Height 2 cm

唇口，束颈，溜肩，鼓腹，平底，圈足。盛药器具。

邢窑出品。1958 年西安市韩森寨出土。

陕西医史博物馆藏

The medicine container has a lip-shaped mouth rim, a contracted neck, a sloping shoulder, a globular body, a flat bottom and a circular foot. The bottle was a production of the Xing kiln, unearthed in Hansenzhai, Xi'an, Shaanxi Province, in the year 1958.

Preserved in Shaanxi Museum of Medical History

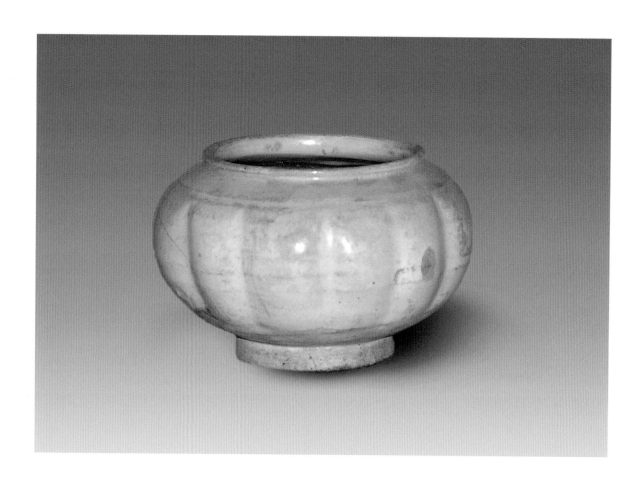

白瓷药罐

唐

瓷质

口径 9 厘米，底径 6.7 厘米，通高 8.4 厘米，重 300 克

White Porcelain Gallipot

Tang Dynasty

Porcelain

Mouth Diameter 9 cm/ Bottom Diameter 6.7 cm/ Height 8.4 cm/ Weight 300 g

唇口，瓜棱腹，圈足，白釉泛青，施釉不到底。医药器具。腹部有裂痕。2002 年入藏。陕西省西安市古玩市场征集。

陕西医史博物馆藏

This gallipot, a medical appliance, has a lip-shaped mouth, a pumpkin-shaped belly and a ring foot. It is covered with white glaze with blue-green tints while its bottom is left unglazed. Cracks can be seen on its belly. It was collected from Xi'an Antique Market, Shaanxi Province, in 2002.

Preserved in Shaanxi Museum of Medical History

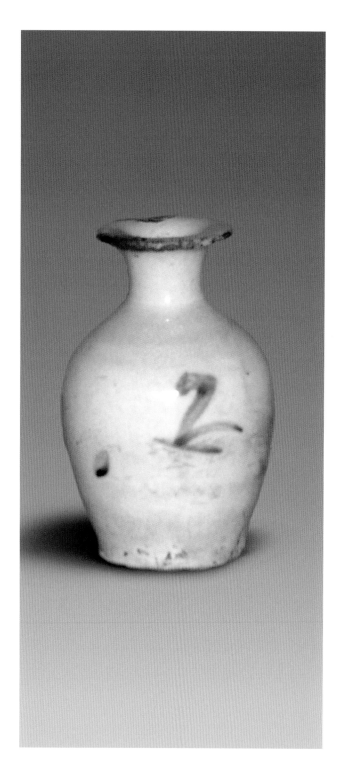

白瓷药瓶

唐

瓷质

口径 3.6 厘米，底径 4 厘米，高 6.5 厘米，重 50 克

White Porcelain Medicine Bottle

Tang Dynasty

Porcelain

Mouth Diameter 3.6 cm/ Bottom Diameter 4 cm/ Height 6.5 cm/ Weight 50 g

小喇叭口，圆肩，圆腹，圈足，通体白釉，绘有小青花。医药器具。口沿残。2001 年 9 月入藏。陕西省西安市古玩市场征集。

陕西医史博物馆藏

With a small trumpet mouth, a round shoulder, a round belly and a ring foot, the bottle is covered with white glaze. On the body was painted a small celadon flower. It was used as a medical appliance. The rim of its mouth was damaged. The bottle was collected from Xi'an Antique Market, Shaanxi Province, in September 2001. Preserved in Shaanxi Museum of Medical History

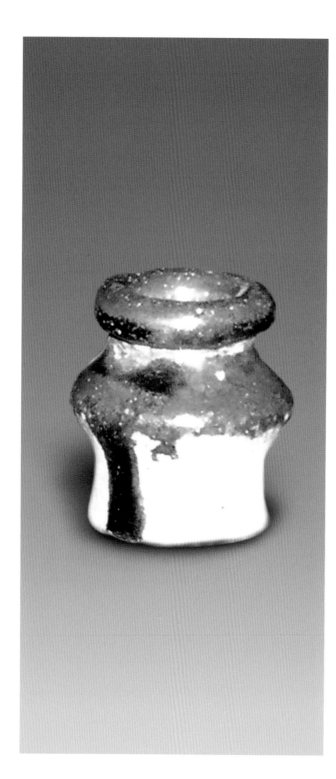

棕釉圆药瓶

唐

瓷质

口径 2.2 厘米，底径 2.3 厘米，高 2.9 厘米，
重 20 克

Brown-glazed Round Medicine Bottle

Tang Dynasty

Porcelain

Mouth Diameter 2.2 cm/ Bottom Diameter 2.3 cm/

Height 2.9 cm/ Weight 20 g

唇口，束颈，折腹，平底，瓶内及瓶外上半部施釉。药具。保存完整。2002 年入藏。陕西省咸阳市征集。

陕西医史博物馆藏

It has a lip-shaped mouth, a contracted neck, an angular belly and a flat bottom. Its upper half, both inside and outside, is coated with glaze. It served as a medical appliance and has been kept in good shape. The bottle was collected from Xianyang, Shaanxi Province, in the year 2002. Preserved in Shaanxi Museum of Medical History

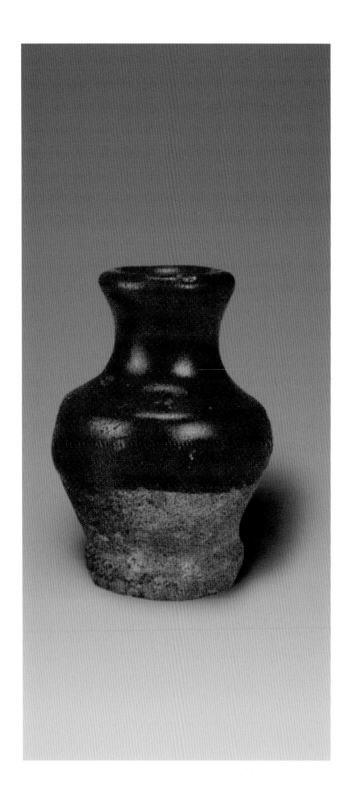

黑釉瓷药瓶

唐

瓷质

口径 1.7 厘米，底径 1.8 厘米，高 4 厘米

Black-glazed Porcelain Medicine Bottle

Tang Dynasty

Porcelain

Mouth Diameter 1.7 cm/ Bottom Diameter 1.8 cm/

Height 4 cm

唇口，长颈，折腹，平底，瓶内与瓶身上部施釉。
盛药器具。陕西旬邑唐代窑址出土。

陕西医史博物馆藏

With the inside wall and the upper part glazed, the bottle has a lip-shaped mouth rim, a long neck, an angular belly and a flat bottom. The bottle served as a medicine container. The bottle was unearthed from the kiln of the Tang Dynasty, Xunyi County, Shaanxi Province.

Preserved in Shaanxi Museum of Medical History

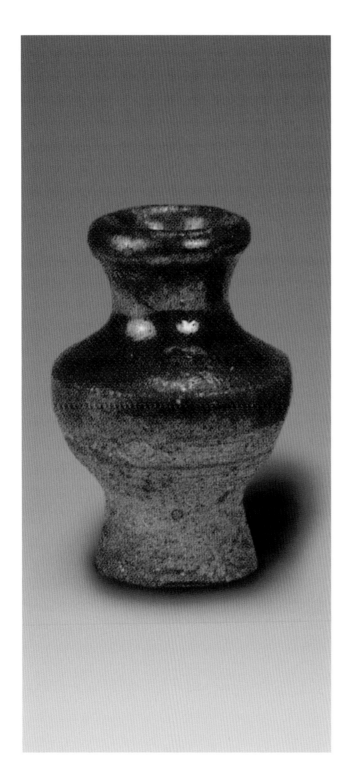

黑釉瓷药瓶

唐

瓷质

口径 1.7 厘米，底径 2.1 厘米，瓶高 4.2 厘米

Black-glazed Porcelain Medicine Bottle

Tang Dynasty

Porcelain

Mouth Diameter 1.7 cm/ Bottom Diameter 2.1 cm/

Height 4.2 cm

唇口，束颈，折腹，平底，瓶内与瓶身上半部分施釉。盛药器具。陕西旬邑唐代窑址出土。

陕西医史博物馆藏

With a lip-shaped mouth rim, a contracted neck, an angular belly stomach and a flat bottom, this bottle was glazed on the upper part and the inside wall, and was used as a medicine container. The bottle was unearthed from the kiln of the Tang Dynasty, Xunyi County, Shaanxi Province.

Preserved in Shaanxi Museum of Medical History

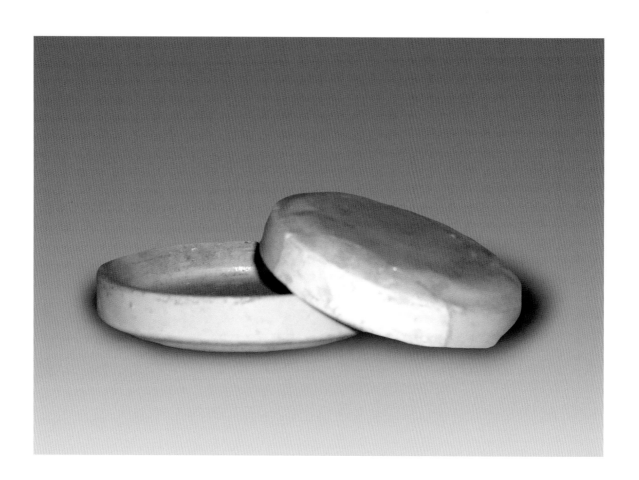

白瓷药盒

唐

瓷质

盖口径 8.5 厘米，底径 9.5 厘米，通高 2.5 厘米，重 500 克

White-glazed Medicine Box

Tang Dynasty

Porcelain

Lid: Mouth Diameter 8.5 cm/ Bottom Diameter 9.5 cm/ Height 2.5 cm/ Weight 500 g

子母口，直腹，平底，白瓷，无纹饰。贮药器。

有修补。陕西省西安市何家村征集。

陕西医史博物馆藏

With a buckle lid, a straight belly and a flat
bottom, the plain box is coated with white glaze.
It was utilized for storing medicine and marks of
touch-up coating can be found on it. The bottle
was collected from Hejia Village, Xi'an, Shaanxi
Province.

Preserved in Shaanxi Museum of Medical History

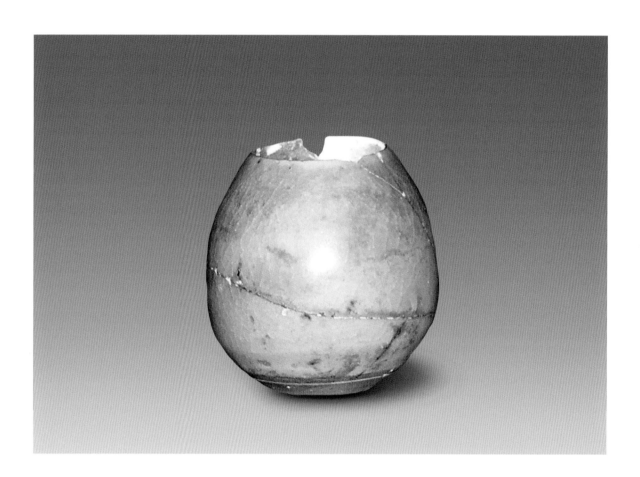

拔火罐

唐

瓷质

口径 2 厘米，底径 2 厘米，通高 4.1 厘米，重 2300 克

Cupping Cup

Tang Dynasty

Porcelain

Mouth Diameter 2 cm/ Bottom Diameter 2cm/ Height 4.1cm/ Weight 2,300g

敛口，圆腹，平底，豆绿色薄细小。医药器具，
有修补。陕西省铜川市征集。

陕西医史博物馆藏

This cup is coated with light green glaze in a
fine and thin fashion. It has a contracted mouth,
a round belly and a flat bottom. It was used
as a medical appliance and marks of touch-
up coating can be found on it. The cup was
collected from Tongchuan, Shaanxi Province.

Preserved in Shaanxi Museum of Medical History

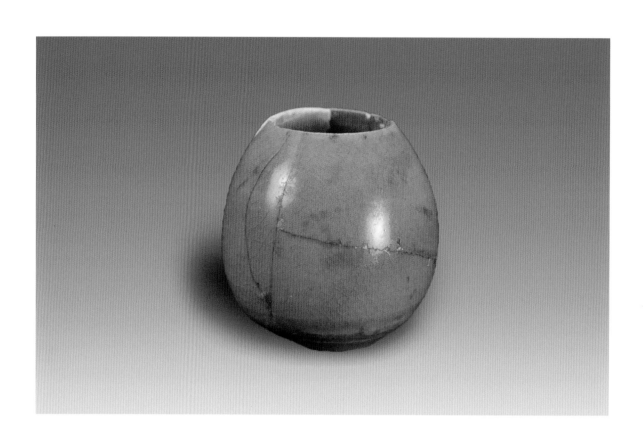

耀瓷拔火罐

唐

瓷质

口径 2.3 厘米，底径 2.1 厘米，高 4.7 厘米

口沿已有残缺。20 世纪 70 年代陕西铜川黄堡唐代窑址出土。

陕西医史博物馆藏

Porcelain Cupping Cup, Yao Ware

Tang Dynasty

Porcelain

Mouth Diameter 2.3 cm/ Bottom Diameter 2.1 cm/ Height 4.7 cm

The rim of the cup's mouth was damaged. The cup was unearthed from the kiln of the Tang Dynasty in Huangbu, Tongchuan, Shaanxi Province, in the 1970s.

Preserved in Shaanxi Museum of Medical History

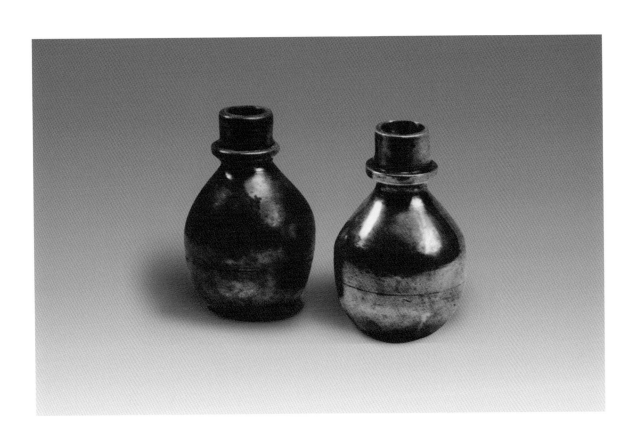

石榴罐

唐

瓷质

口内深 1.3 厘米，孔径 0.4 厘米

圆底，炼丹用器物。1970 年西安市何家村出土。

陕西历史博物馆藏

Pomegranate-shaped Jars

Tang Dynasty

Porcelain

Mouth Depth 1.3 cm/ Hole Diameter 0.4 cm

With round bottoms, the jars were utilized for
Taoist alchemy. They were unearthed in Hejia
Village, Xi'an, Shaanxi Province, in 1970.

Preserved in Shaanxi History Museum

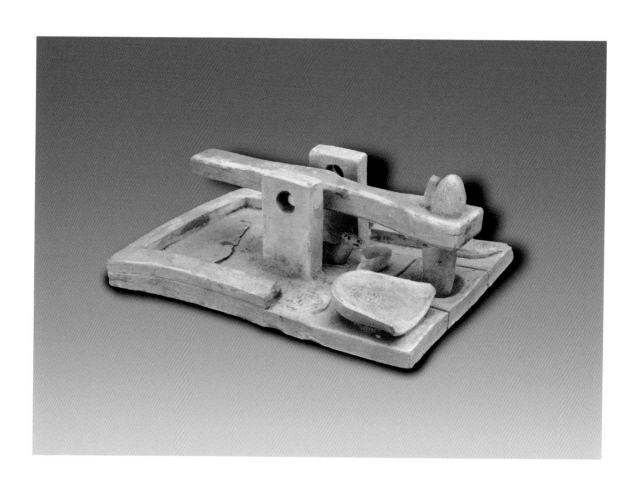

陶舂米机

唐

陶质

长 23.5 厘米，宽 15 厘米，通高 9 厘米

Pottery Rice-thrashing Machine

Tang Dynasty

Pottery

Length 23.5 cm/ Width 15 cm/ Height 9 cm

陶制舂米机的模型。舂米棒安装在长柄的一端，下置臼槽，长柄中间用架子支撑。舂米机下塑有一只温驯的小犬，小犬前置食槽。在舂米机左右两侧各置簸箕、笤帚。

陕西省昭陵博物馆藏

This item is a model of pottery rice-thrashing machine model. In the middle of the long handle, a supportive frame was constructed. A rice-thrashing stick was installed at one end of the long handle, under which is a mortar. With a crib put in front, there is a docile doggie posed under the trashing machine, where a winnowing fan and a broom were respectively placed at each side.

Preserved in Zhaoling Museum, Shaanxi Province

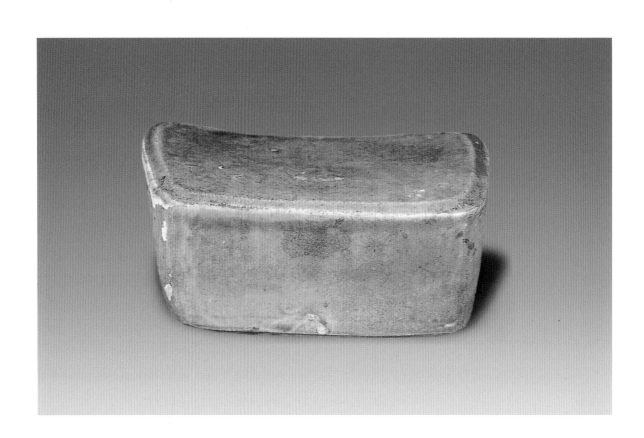

黄釉脉枕

唐

瓷质

长 15 厘米，宽 8 厘米，高 7.2 厘米

诊脉用。

上海中医药博物馆藏

Yellow-glazed Wrist Cushion

Tang Dynasty

Porcelain

Length 15 cm/ Width 8 cm/ Height 7.2 cm

This cushion covered by yellow glaze is designed for the purpose of pause-taking.

Preserved in Shanghai Museum of Traditional Chinese Medicine

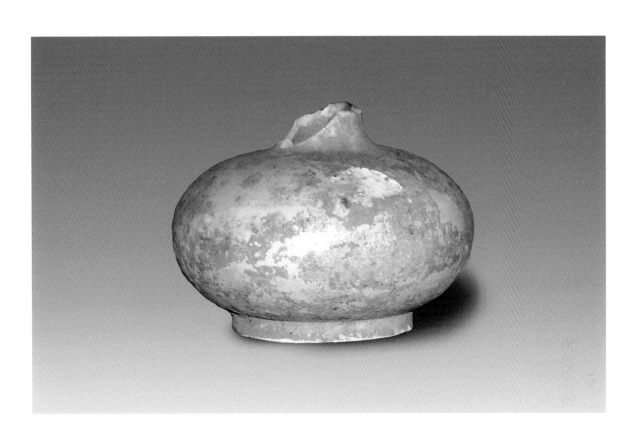

白瓷瓶

唐

瓷质

口径 3 厘米，底径 6.6 厘米，通高 8.5 厘米，重 300 克

圆腹，圈足，白瓷。生活用器。口残。

陕西医史博物馆藏

White Porcelain Vase

Tang Dynasty

Porcelain

Mouth Diameter 3 cm/ Bottom Diameter 6.6 cm/ Height 8.5 cm/ Weight 300 g

The white vase is characterized with a round belly and a ring foot. The mouth was damaged. It was used as a household utensil.

Preserved in Shaanxi Museum of Medical History

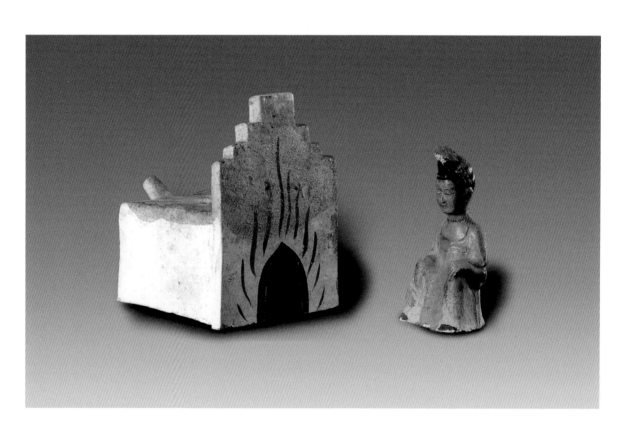

彩釉灶和司灶俑

唐

瓷质

俑：高 11 厘米

灶：长 14 厘米，宽 12 厘米，高 16 厘米

Colour-glazed Cooking Stove and Fire-guarding Figurine

Tang Dynasty

Porcelain

Figurine: Height 11 cm

Cooking Stove: Length 14 cm/ Width 12 cm/ Height 16 cm

陶灶为长方形，其上置一锅，灶后带有烟囱，灶门为半椭圆形，灶膛里的红色火苗扑出灶门外。灶前坐一高髻、圆脸的中年妇女，上穿方领低胸窄袖衫，下着长裙，背上披一小方巾，两腿弯曲，双膝并拢，左手置于膝上，右手轻轻贴于小腿，似正在静观灶膛中的火势，以待添柴。造型自然，逼真，优美。

陕西省昭陵博物馆藏

A wok is located on the top of the rectangular cooking stove and a chimney stands at the back. Signs of red flames are seemingly coming out from the semioval stove door. In front of the stove sits a middleaged woman with a round face and updo hair style. She is wearing a low-cut, square collared and narrow sleeved blouse and a long skirt, with a small square scarf covering her back. The woman bends her legs with both knees close to each other, and has her left hand placed on the knee, right hand attached to the shins. she seems to be watching over the fire in the stove, ready to add firewood if necessary. The whole vessel looks natural, vivid and beautiful.

Preserved in Zhaoling Museum, Shaanxi Province

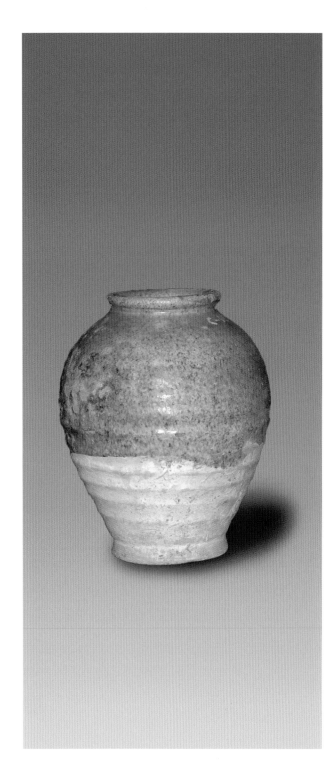

黄釉罐

唐

瓷质

口径 6 厘米，底径 6.4 厘米，通高 14 厘米，重 400 克

Yellow-glazed Jar

Tang Dynasty

Porcelain

Mouth Diameter 6 cm/ Bottom Diameter 6.4 cm/

Height 14 cm/ Weight 400 g

圆唇，鼓腹，平底，腹下半部无釉，周身粗弦纹。

盛贮器。完整无损。陕西省西安市何家村征集。

陕西医史博物馆藏

With a round lip-shaped mouth, a swelling belly and a flat bottom, the jar is coated with glaze only on its upper half and its whole body is decorated with bold bowstring patterns. It served as a containing and storing vessel, and has been kept intact. It was collected from Hejia Village, Xi'an, Shaanxi Province.

Preserved in Shaanxi Museum of Medical History

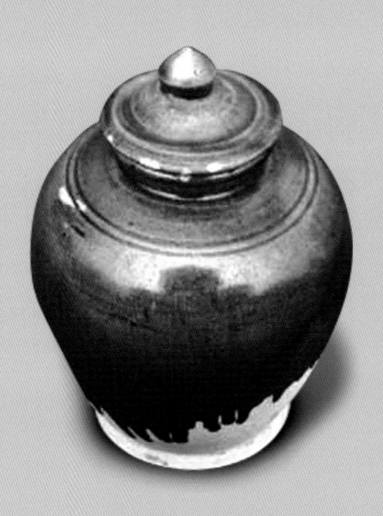

黄釉陶罐

唐

瓷质

外口径 6.63 厘米，腹径 12.7 厘米，底径 8.8 厘米，通高 18.6 厘米，腹深 14.2 厘米，重 715 克

腹部上鼓下敛，圈足。带盖陶罐，盛物容器，生活用品。

广东中医药博物馆藏

Yellow-glazed Pottery Jar

Tang dynasty

Pottery

Outer Mouth Diameter 6.63 cm/ Belly Diameter 12.7 cm/ Bottom Diameter 8.8 cm/ Height 18.6 cm/ Depth 14.2 cm/ Weight 715 g

The jar has a lid, a ring foot and a swelling belly which gradually tapers downwards. It served as a household utensil.

Preserved in Guangdong Chinese Medicine Museum

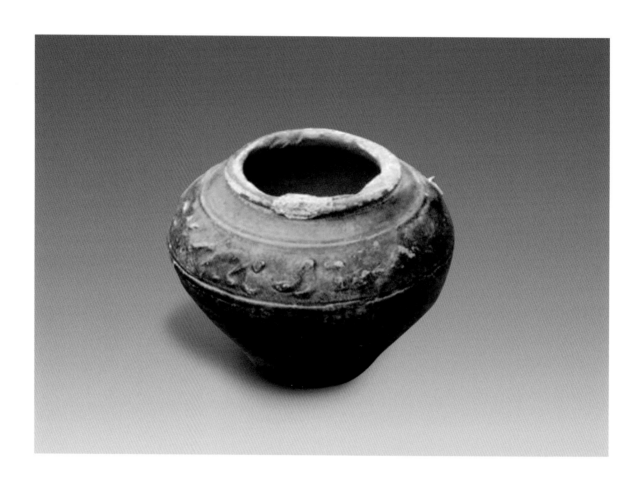

绿釉陶罐

唐

陶质

外口径 8.2 厘米，腹径 11 厘米，底径 6.6 厘米，通高 11.6 厘米，腹深 10.8 厘米

Green-glazed Pottery Jar

Tang dynasty

Pottery

Outer Mouth Diameter 8.2 cm/ Belly Diameter 11 cm/ Bottom Diameter 6.6 cm/ Height 11.6 cm/ Depth 10.8 cm

陶质，平口，口沿外侈，鼓腹，腹有弦纹，腹上部堆花纹，平底，底边沿外展。盛物用。

广东中医药博物馆藏

The jar has a flat mouth with its rim flared, a swelling belly decorated with string pattern, and a flat bottom whose edge extends outward. Flower patterns emerge on its upper belly. The jar was used as a container.

Preserved in Guangdong Chinese Medicine Museum

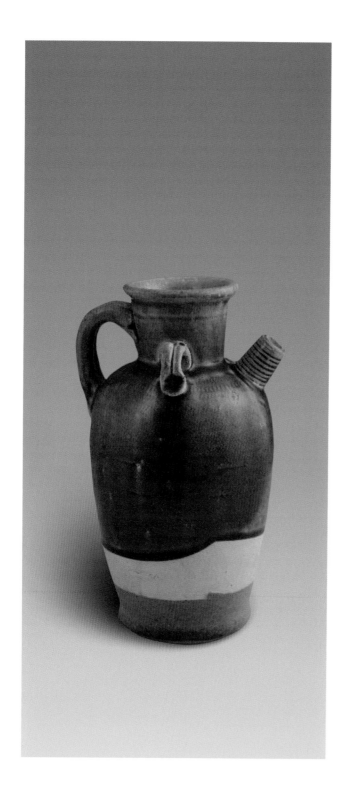

黄釉执壶

唐

瓷质

口径 9 厘米，高 36 厘米

Yellow-glazed Ewer (Porcelain Pot)

Tang Dynasty

Porcelain

Mouth Diameter 9 cm/ Height 36 cm

侈口，直斜颈，溜肩，短直流与半环状提梁相对，

双耳，斜腹，平底，圈足。用于盛装露水等。

北京御生堂中医药博物馆藏

The pot has a widely flared mouth, a straight neck, a narrow and incline shoulder, two ears, an inclined belly, a flat bottom and a ring feet. The short and straight spout is opposite to semi ring-shaped handle. It was used for storing clew.

Preserved in Chinese Medicine Museum of Beijing Yu Sheng Tang Drugstore

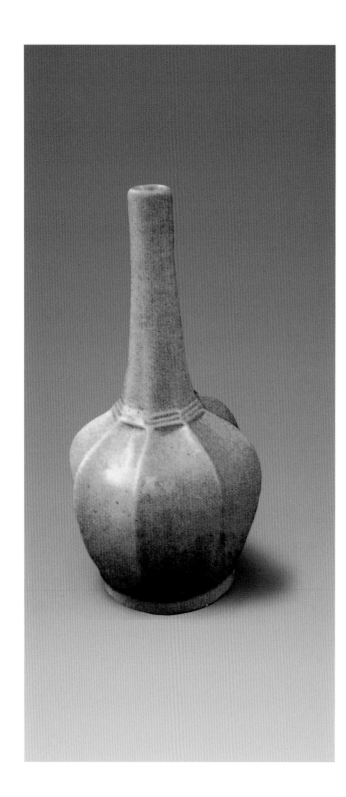

八棱净水瓶

唐

瓷质

底径 10.2 厘米，高 21.4 厘米

Octagonal Vase for Holding Holy Water

Tang dynasty

Porcelain

Bottom Diameter 10.2 cm/ Height 21.4 cm

圆口，长颈，圆腹，颈底部饰三周台阶形八方

弦纹。肩腹部竖向凸饰八条棱线，圈足。秘色瓷。

1987 年陕西扶风法门寺出土。

陕西省法门寺博物馆藏

With eight vertical protruding chine lines
molded from the shoulder to the abdomen, this
vase has a round rim, a long neck with step-
shaped string patterns pointed to the eight
compass directions, a globular abdomen, and
a circular foot. This vase is a porcelain ware
of secret colour. It was unearthed in Famen
Temple in Fufeng County, Shaanxi Province, in
the year 1987.

Preserved in Famen Temple Museum, Shaanxi
Province

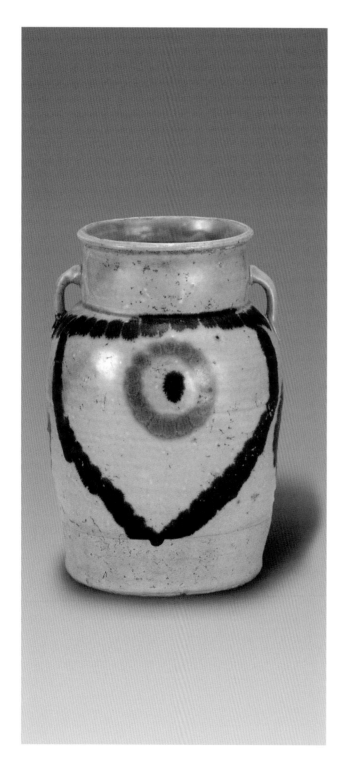

青釉褐绿点彩双耳罐

唐

瓷质

口径 8.8 厘米，高 17 厘米

Celadon Jar with Double Ears and Breen Stippling

Tang Dynasty

Porcelain

Mouth Diameter 8.8 cm/ Height 17 cm

直口，粗颈，削肩，直筒形腹，底内凹。颈肩连接处置对称泥条双系。胎灰黄，施青黄色釉，不及底。腹部两面各施以褐彩点，中心再点一褐彩点。两外圈之间各以一中心点蓝彩的褐圈填饰。图案简洁明快，具有浓郁的西亚风格。1978 年扬州市汶河路出土。

扬州博物馆藏

The jar has a straight mouth, a stout neck, a sloping shoulder, a straight belly and a concave bottom with two symmetrical ears at the junction of the neck and the shoulder on either side. The greyish-yellow body is covered with celadon-yellow glaze, but the lower part and the bottom are left unglazed. Both sides of the belly are enameled with brown speckles, and one such speckle is found at its centre as well. Between two outer circles is painted a brown ring around a blue dot. This pattern looks concise and vibrant, revealing a rich West Asian style. The vessel was unearthed from Wenhe Road, Yangzhou, Jiangsu Province, in 1978.

Preserved in Yangzhou Museum

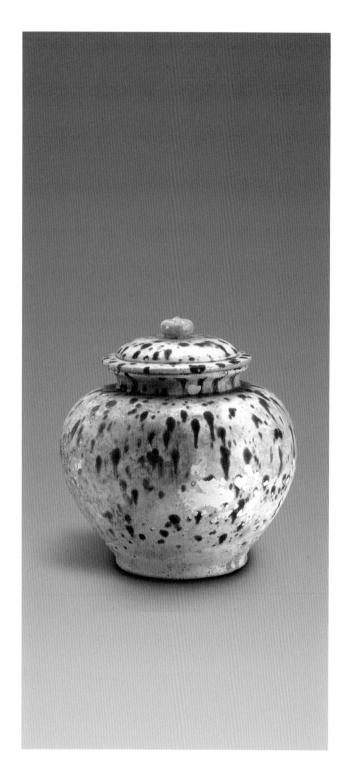

白釉蓝彩盖罐

唐

瓷质

口径 10.4 厘米，通高 17.8 厘米

Covered White-glazed Jar with Blue Spots

Tang Dynasty

Porcelain

Mouth Diameter 10.4 cm/ Height 17.8 cm

侈口，束颈，鼓腹，下腹渐收，平底。上置扁平盖，扁圆钮。胎白且细腻。满施白釉，色微泛黄，通体以蓝釉洒点成自然的纹饰，如潇潇雨下，颇具特色。1974 年扬州市城北乡红星村出土。

扬州博物馆藏

The jar has a wide flared mouth, a contracted neck, a bulging belly, the lower part of which gradually tapers down, and a flat bottom. It has a flat lid with an oblate knob. The fine white body is covered with white glaze with a tint of yellow. The whole jar is decorated evenly with blue-glazed speckles in the form of rain drops. It was unearthed from Hongxing Village, Chengbei Town, Yangzhou, Jiangsu Province in 1974.

Preserved in Yangzhou Museum

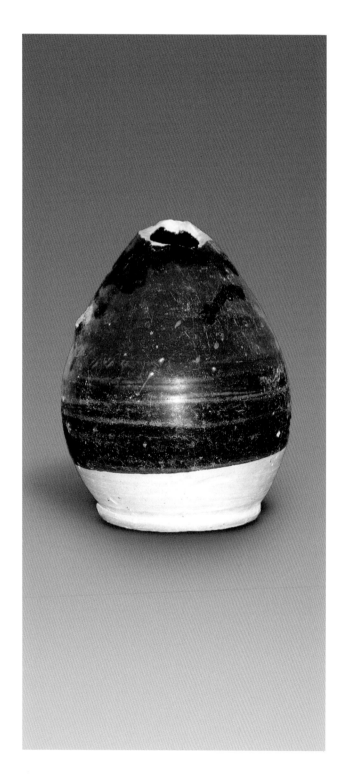

黑瓷瓶

唐

瓷质

口径 10 厘米，底径 13 厘米，通高 24 厘米，

重 2150 克

Black-glazed Bottle

Tang dynasty

Porcelain

Mouth Diameter 10 cm/ Bottom Diameter 13 cm/

Height 24 cm/ Weight 2,150 g

塔状，圈足，黑釉，下腹和底无釉白胎。盛贮器。
口残，把残。

陕西医史博物馆藏

The bottle has a ring foot and is tower-shaped.
Its white body is coated with black glaze, with
its lower belly and bottom left unglazed. It
served as a container. Its mouth and handle
were damaged.

Preserved in Shaanxi Museum of Medical History

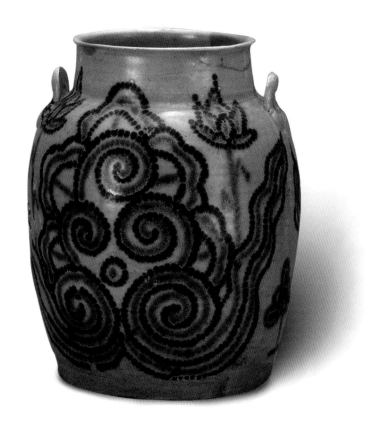

青釉褐绿点彩云纹双耳罐

唐

瓷质

口径 16.3 厘米，底径 19.5 厘米，高 29.8 厘米

Double-eared Celadon Jar with Breen Stippling Cloud Design

Tang Dynasty

Porcelain

Mouth Diameter 16.3 cm/ Bottom Diameter 19.5 cm/ Height 29.8 cm

直口，卷唇，高颈，鼓腹，平底。肩部置对称扁环形双系，系上饰云纹和"王"字。胎为米黄色，通体施青黄色釉，器身布满纹饰，以褐、绿两色相间的大小斑点组成联珠状卷云图案，每组之间绘莲叶和莲花纹。长沙窑制品。1974年扬州市唐城遗址出土。

扬州博物馆藏

The jar has a straight mouth with a rolled rim, a tall neck, a swelling belly and a flat bottom. Double symmetrical oval rings, decorated with cloud patterns and the Chinese character "Wang" (a king), emerge on its shoulder. The entire off-white body is coated with celadon-yellow glaze and decorated with motifs. The string-bead cloud design is made up of brown and green speckles. Between groups of cloud design are painted lotus patterns. The vessel was made in the Changsha kiln and was unearthed from the city ruins of the Tang Dynasty, Yangzhou, Jiangsu Province, in the year 1974.

Preserved in Yangzhou Museum

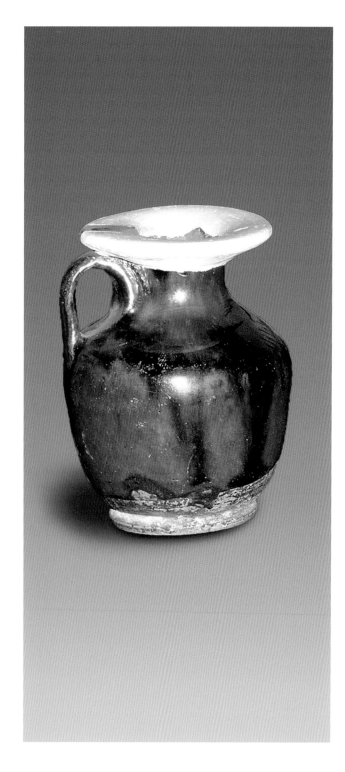

单耳黑釉陶瓶

唐

陶质

口径 4.5 厘米，底径 3.4 厘米，通高 7 厘米，

重 90 克

Black-glazed Pottery Bottle with Single Ear

Tang Dynasty

Pottery

Mouth Diameter 4.5 cm/ Bottom Diameter 3.4 cm/

Height 7 cm/ Weight 90 g

喇叭形口，折肩，口沿与肩处有一手把，圈足。黑釉。容器。口沿有残，已修复。陕西省西安市征集。

陕西医史博物馆藏

The black-glazed bottle has a trumpet mouth, an angular shoulder and a ring foot, with a handle between the mouth rim and the shoulder. It served as a container. Its mouth rim was damaged and has been restored later. It was collected from Xi'an, Shaanxi Province.

Preserved in Shaanxi Museum of Medical History

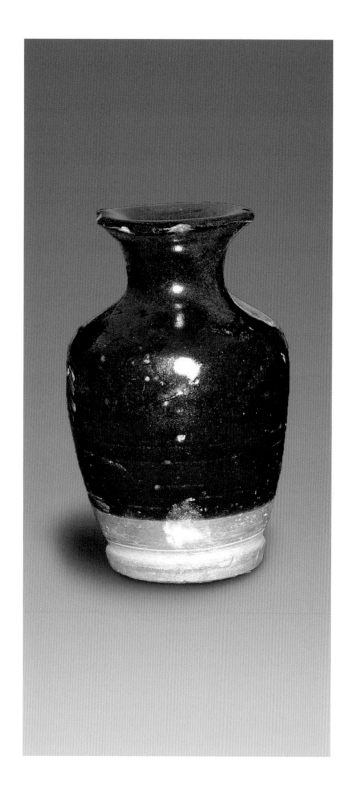

黑釉陶瓶

唐

陶质

口径 4.1 厘米，底径 4 厘米，通高 9.1 厘米，
重 1000 克

Black-glazed Pottery Vase

Tang Dynasty

Pottery

Mouth Diameter 4.1 cm/ Bottom Diameter 4 cm/

Height 9.1 cm/ Weight 1,000 g

喇叭形口，折肩，斜腹，圈足，下五分之一处
为白胎。容器。完整无损。陕西省西安市征集。

陕西医史博物馆藏

The vase is glazed black, except the part above
the bottom, about one fifth of it, revealing its
white body. It is featured with a flared mouth,
an angular shoulder, a sloping belly and a ring
foot. This vessel, still in perfect condition, was
collected from Xi'an, Shaanxi Province.

Preserved in Shaanxi Museum of Medical History

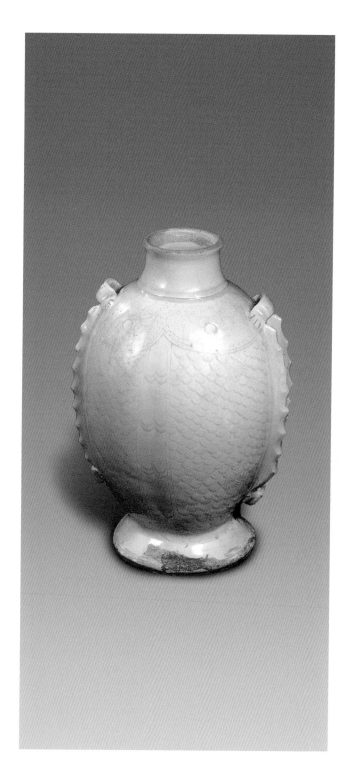

邢窑白釉双鱼背瓶

唐

瓷质

口径 4.9 厘米，底径 9.5 厘米，高 21 厘米

White-glazed Flask in the Shape of Double Fish Backs, Xing Ware

Tang Dynasty

Porcelain

Mouth Diameter 4.9 cm/ Bottom Diameter 9.5 cm/

Height 21 cm

胎洁白细腻而致密，通体施白釉，口缘及足部
露胎，釉色白中闪青。造型呈双鱼跃起状，鱼
头为瓶的口、颈、肩部，身为瓶身，尾为瓶之
圈足。瓶口外侈，腹部扁圆，圈足外撇，瓶身
饰满鱼鳞纹，两侧堆塑双排鱼鳍纹。上、下均
有环形系，圈足置孔，便于穿系提携。

河北博物院藏

The body of this flask is of smooth and dense texture. Except its mouth rim and foot, the flask is coated with white glaze with a cyan shine. The flask is in the shape of two leaping fish. The fish heads serve as the flask's mouth, neck and shoulder, the fish tail as its ring foot and the fish body as the belly of the flask. It has a trumpet mouth, an oblate belly, and a flared ring foot, with its body overlaid with fish-scale patterns, and the sides moulded with two rows of fish-fin. The rings at the four ends of the fish-fins and the holes on the ring foot are designed for ease of hanging or carrying if fastened to a cord.

Preserved in Hebei Museum

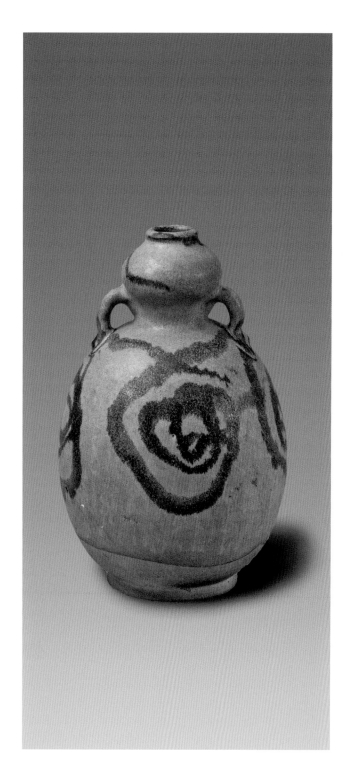

灰釉斑彩葫芦瓶

唐

瓷质

口径 3.5 厘米，底径 9.5 厘米，高 24.6 厘米

Gourd-shaped Flask with Coloured Stripes on Ash Glaze

Tang Dynasty

Porcelain

Mouth Diameter 3.5 cm/ Bottom Diameter 9.5 cm/

Height 24.6 cm

郊县窑产品。胎体厚重，色白。施灰釉不到底。器呈葫芦形，小口，平底，附双耳。腹部饰黑色斑彩，似空中团云状，自然飘浮，色彩醒目。唐郊县窑花袖瓷，其艺术特色是在黑釉、黄釉、天蓝釉上饰以天蓝或月白色的斑点。这种釉上彩斑点是用与底色不同的釉料随意洒刷上的，烧成后自然流淌，变幻多端。

青岛市博物馆藏

This flask was produced in the suburban kiln of the Tang Dynasty. It has a thick and white body, a small mouth, a flat bottom and a pair of ears. It is ash-glazed except its lower part and bottom. Its belly is decorated with black stripes resembling masses of naturally floating clouds in distinctive colours. The artistic characteristic of this fancy glazed porcelain is embodied in the light blue specks on the black, yellow and sapphire glazed ground. Glazes different from its background were randomly sprinkled on the body before it was fired, resulting in a natural and changeful style.

Preserved in Qingdao Municipal Museum

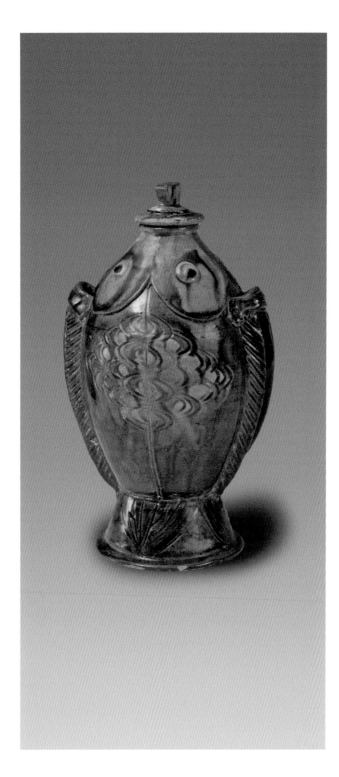

三彩陶双鱼瓶

唐

陶质

口径 4.1 厘米，通高 24.5 厘米

Tricolour Pottery Flask in the Shape of Double-fish

Tang Dynasty

Pottery

Mouth Diameter 4.1 cm/ Height 24.5 cm

小口，深腹，高圈足，圆盖方钮。器身塑双鱼形，嘴、眼、胸鳍、鳞、尾逼真，或凸起，或刻画并施以黄、绿、赭彩，浓淡适宜。盖钮有圆孔，两侧鱼鳍作槽状，上有横贯耳，下与圈足圆相通，可系绳，便于携带。青州市出土。

山东博物馆藏

The flask is featured with a small mouth, a deep belly, a tall ring foot and a round lid with a square knob. It is sculpted into the shape of double fish with life-like mouths, eyes, fins, scales and tail. Some parts are protruding, while others carved and painted in yellow, green and reddish brown. The tapped hole on the flask knob, the loop ears and the bilateral groove-shaped fins connecting the ears and the ring foot are designed for ease of hanging and carrying if fastened to a cord. It was unearthed in Qingzhou, Shandong Province.

Preserved in Shandong Museum

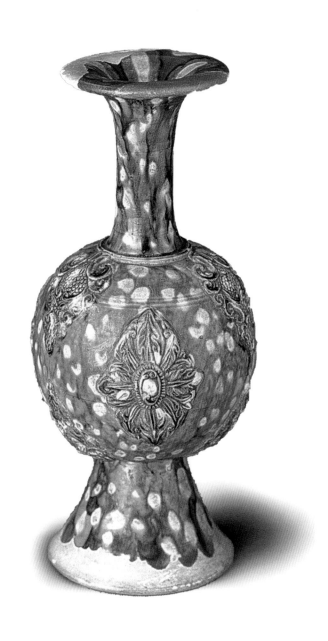

三彩贴花瓶

唐

瓷质

口径 7.7 厘米，高 24.2 厘米

敞口，细长颈，喇叭足，除圈足外施黄、绿、白三彩釉斑点。

山西省博物馆藏

Tricolour Vase Decorated with Decal Flowers

Tang Dynasty

Porcelain

Mouth Diameter 7.7 cm/ Height 24.2 cm

The vase has a flared mouth, a long narrow neck, and a trumpet foot. The whole vase is glazed with Tricolour speckles of yellow, green and white, except the ring foot.

Preserved in Shanxi Museum

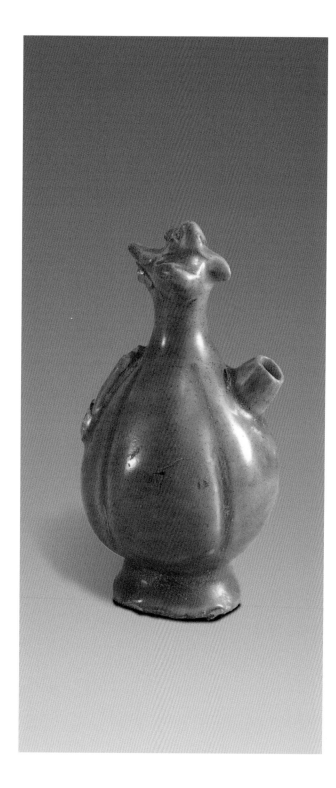

凤头壶

唐

瓷质

高 10 厘米

Phoenix-head Pot

Tang Dynasty

Porcelain

Height 10 cm

器上部作凤头状，腹下垂，作瓜棱状，短嘴，把残，满青釉。

浙江省文物考古研究所藏

This pot has a short mouth with the handle broken. Its upper part is in the shape of a phoenix head, and its droopy belly resembles a melon with incised lines. It is fully coated with celadon.

Preserved in Institute of Cultural Relics and Archaeology of Zhejiang Province

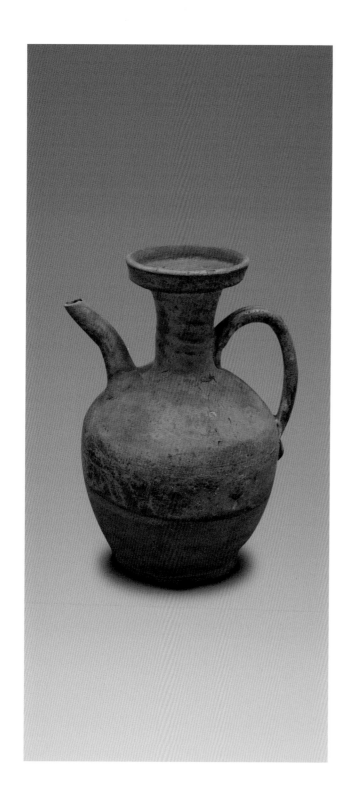

壶

唐

瓷质

腹径 12.5 厘米，高 20 厘米

Flask

Tang Dynasty

Porcelain

Belly Diameter 12.5 cm/ Height 20 cm

盘口，竹节形颈，鼓腹，平底，环形把，细长形流，施青釉至腹中部，下部露胎。保存完整。由成都考古队调拨。

成都中医药大学中医药传统文化博物馆藏

Attached with a ring handle and a slender spout, the flask is also characterized with a bulging belly, a flat bottom, a disk-shaped mouth and a neck in the shape of bamboo segments. It is glazed with celadon from the top to the middle of the belly, with the lower part left unglazed. The pot which was allocated from the Chengdu Municipal Archaeological Team is still in good shape.

Preserved in Museum of Traditional Chinese Medicine Culture, Chengdu University of Traditional Chinese Medicine

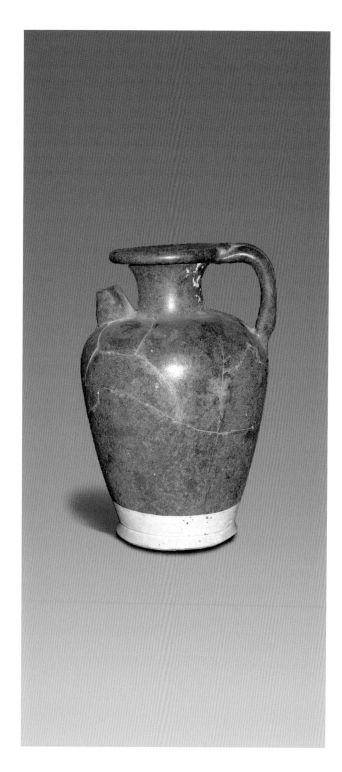

陶壶

唐

陶质

口径 8.8 厘米，底径 9.4 厘米，通高 21 厘米，
重 1000 克

Pottery Flask

Tang Dynasty

Pottery

Mouth Diameter 8.8 cm/ Bottom Diameter 9.4 cm/

Height 21 cm/ Weight 1,000 g

喇叭口，口沿与肩处有一把手，肩部有一短流，圆肩，斜腹。盛贮器。有修补。陕西省西安市征集。

陕西医史博物馆藏

This pottery flask has an oblique belly and a trumpet mouth, whose rim is connected by a handle to its round shoulder where a short spout protrudes. It was used as a storage vessel, and marks of restoration could be found on it. The flask was collected in Xi'an, Shaanxi Province.

Preserved in Shaanxi Museum of Medical History

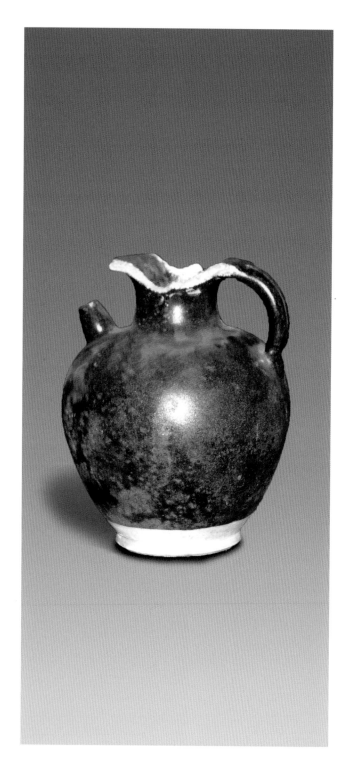

黑釉壶

唐

瓷质

口径 8 厘米，底径 7.5 厘米，通高 16.5 厘米，
重 800 克

Black-glazed Pot

Tang Dynasty

Porcelain

Mouth Diameter 8 cm/ Bottom Diameter 7.5 cm/

Height 16.5 cm/ Weight 800 g

喇叭口，直颈，口腹之间有把，肩处有一壶嘴。

盛贮器，生活用器。口残。陕西省鄠邑区征集。

陕西医史博物馆藏

This pot, a household utensil for storage, has a damaged flared mouth, and an upright neck. Its mouth, and belly are connected by a handle, and on its shoulder is a spout. It was collected from Huyi District, Shaanxi Province.

Preserved in Shaanxi Museum of Medical History

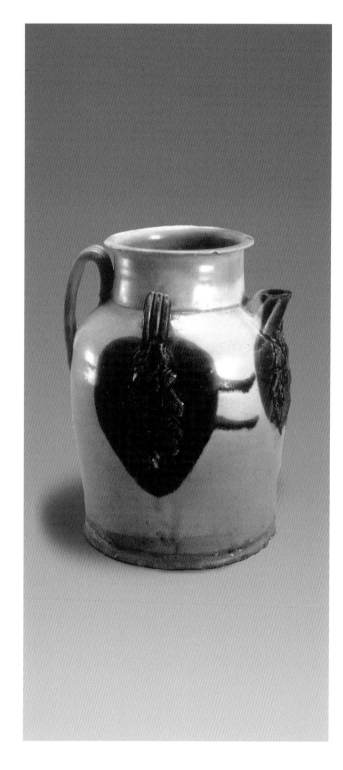

青釉褐彩巾饰人物狮纹壶

唐

瓷质

口径 9.7 厘米，底径 12.6 厘米，高 18.6 厘米

Brown-Specked Celadon Ewer Decorated with Figure and Lion Patterns

Tang Dynasty

Porcelain

Mouth Diameter 9.7 cm/ Bottom Diameter 12.6 cm/

Height 18.6 cm

壶口沿微撇，直颈，斜肩，筒形腹，平底。肩部置八棱形短流，三泥条宽鋬，两侧对贴环形系。双系下各贴一模印吹笛人物，流下贴一狮纹，均覆以叶形褐彩斑块。胎色灰黄，施青黄色釉，釉色纯正滋润。长沙窑制品。1978年扬州市仓巷出土。

扬州博物馆藏

The ewer has a mouth with a flared rim, an upright neck, a sloping shoulder, a barrel-shaped belly and a flat bottom. An octagonal short spout and a handle made of three clay strips are placed on the shoulder, while a pair of rings flanks the shoulder. Below each of the rings is stuck a stamped figure playing the flute, and below the spout is a lion pattern. The rings, the figure, the spout and the lion are all covered with leave-shaped brown patches. The greyish yellow body of the ewer is coated with blue-yellow glaze, which is pure and mellow. It was produced in a kiln in Changsha, and was unearthed in Cangxiang, Yangzhou, Jiangsu Province, in the year 1978.

Preserved in Yangzhou Museum

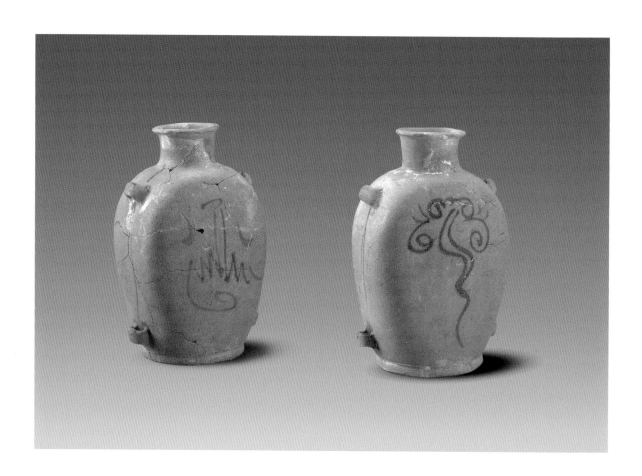

青釉绿彩阿拉伯文扁壶

唐

瓷质

口径 6 厘米，通高 17 厘米

Flat Celadon Flask Incised with Arabic Letters

Tang Dynasty

Porcelain

Mouth Diameter 6 cm/ Height 17 cm

壶唇口微撇，直颈，溜肩，橄榄形扁平腹，平底。壶身两侧各有双耳，为背水穿带用。壶身通体施青绿色釉，一面用绿彩绘有长脚花云气纹，一面用绿彩绘有古阿拉伯文"真主最伟大"铭文。此壶的造型，铭文和纹样具有浓郁的西亚风格，而壶的产地在中国长沙窑。这是一件反映唐代中西文化合璧的重要信物。1980年出土于扬州东风砖瓦厂唐代土坑木棺墓中。

扬州博物馆藏

This flask has a slightly flared mouth with a lip-like rim, an upright neck, a sloping shoulder and a flat bottom. Its oblate belly is in the shape of an olive and is flanked by a pair of ears, which are used to tie cords for the ease of carrying water. It is fully covered with cyan glaze, and on one side of the body are painted patterns of floating clouds with a far-extending tail, and on the other side is incised the ancient Arabic inscription "Allahu Akbar" in green. Though produced in Changsha kiln of China, it shows strong features of West Asia in its style, inscription and design. It provides sound evidences of the integration of the Chinese and Western cultures in the Tang Dynasty. It was unearthed in a wooden coffin of a tomb pit of the Tang Dynasty in Dongfeng brick kiln in Yangzhou, Jiangsu Province.

Preserved in Yangzhou Museum

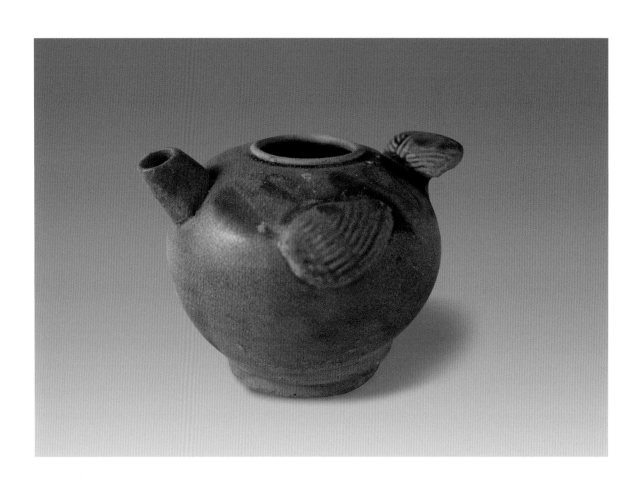

长沙铜官窑青釉彩绘鸟形壶

唐

瓷质

口径 3.6 厘米，底径 5.2 厘米，高 9.3 厘米

Bird-shaped Celadon Ewer with Painted Designs, Tongguan Ware

Tang Dynasty

Porcelain

Mouth Diameter 3.6 cm/ Bottom Diameter 5.2 cm/ Height 9.3 cm

小口，瓜棱形圆腹，平底。壶肩部鸟首为流，
扁形鸟尾为把，肩的两侧雕饰鸟翅。流首、尾部、
翅肩等地方有褐、绿两色釉斑，难得的是呈现
红色彩斑。全身施青釉，青釉中闪微黄，开小
纹片。沙底无釉。该造型较为少见，是长沙窑
的佳作。

吴德蔚藏

This ewer is characterized with a small mouth,
a melon-shaped belly and a flat bottom. The
bird's head on the ewer's shoulder is the spout,
and the bird's flat tail is the handle. A pair of
wings flanks its shoulder, and on the head of
the spout, the tail, the wings and the shoulder
can be seen brown and green glazed speckles.
The red speckles that the ewer carries are rarely
found elsewhere. It is fully celadon-glazed with
slight hints of yellow and small crackles except
for its bottom. With its unique designs, it is a
fine piece of work produced in Changsha kiln.
Collected by Wu Dewei

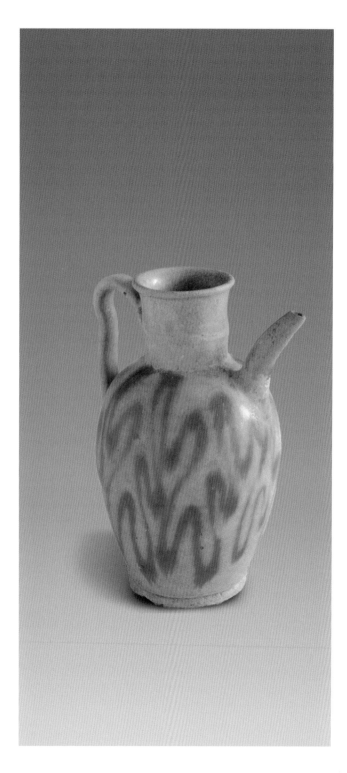

长沙铜官窑绿彩青釉执壶

唐

瓷质

口径 8.3 厘米，底径 9.7 厘米，高 16.6 厘米

Celadon Ewer with Green Paints, Tongguan Ware

Tang Dynasty

Porcelain

Mouth Diameter 8.3 cm/ Bottom Diameter 9.7 cm/

Height 16.6 cm

侈口，卷唇，长直颈，溜肩，腹下部至底渐收，平底。肩至颈上部置扁圆形把，流呈圆筒形。表面施淡青釉，腹部以绿彩画云气纹，线条流畅奔放。长沙铜官窑釉下彩制品，开创了中国陶瓷釉下彩绘之先河。

黄惠边藏

This ewer has a flared mouth with a scrolled rim, a long and upright neck, a sloping shoulder, a tapering belly and a flat bottom. The upper part of its neck is connected to the shoulder by an oblate handle, and its spout is in the shape of a cylinder. The ewer is glazed light greenish blue, and its belly is embellished with green cloud patterns painted in moving and forceful lines. This kind of under-glaze porcelain ware, produced in Tongguan kiln in Changsha, set a precedent in the under-glaze porcelain history in China.

Collected by Huang Huibian

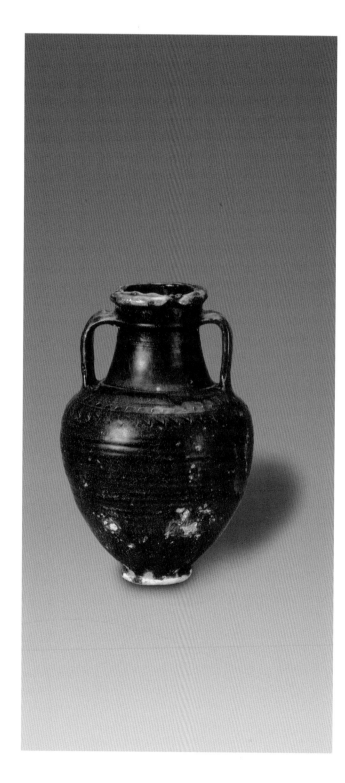

西亚绿釉陶壶

唐

瓷质

口径 9 厘米，底径 10 厘米，高 38 厘米

Green-glazed Pottery Pot of West Asia

Tang Dynasty

Porcelain

Mouth Diameter 9 cm/ Bottom Diameter 10 cm/

Height 38 cm

唇口，高颈，丰肩，鼓腹，腹下渐收，饼形足，底心内凹。上部下方至肩置条形对称双耳。内、外壁均施绿色釉。近底部有底釉，底足微露土黄色胎。通件饰弦纹和水波纹，此器造型硕大，具有鲜明的异域风格，是研究中西交通史的重要实物资料。1965 年扬州市汽车修配厂出土。

扬州博物馆藏

This pot is characterized with a lip-shaped mouth, a long neck, a big shoulder, a pie-shaped foot. The upper part of the and the shoulder are connected by a symmetrical pair of strip-shaped ears. Both the inner and outer walls are coated with green glaze, while the part near the bottom is covered with ground coat paint. The foot reveals a hint of its earthy-yellow body. The pot is fully embellished with grains of string and water ripples. Large in size, the pot, presenting distinct exotic features, provides material data for the study of the history of Sino-foreign communication. It was unearthed from a motor repair factory in Yangzhou, Jiangsu Province, in the year 1965.

Preserved in Yangzhou Museum

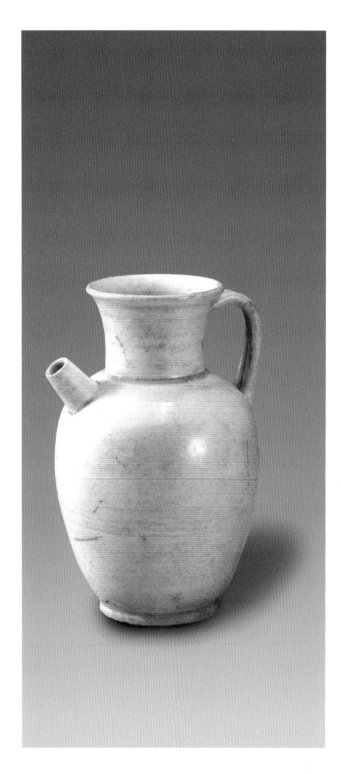

白釉执壶

唐

瓷质

口径 7.5 厘米，底径 6.4 厘米，高 17.3 厘米

White Porcelain Ewer

Tang Dynasty

Porcelain

Mouth Diameter 7.5 cm/ Bottom Diameter 6.4 cm/

Height 17.3 cm

喇叭形口，高颈，斜肩，长圆形腹，腹下部渐收敛，饼形足而底平，颈、肩之间置复合环形柄，相对应处置圆形短流。壶胎骨坚致，修胎规矩，造型端庄，在胎与白釉之间施有护胎釉。此壶系河北邢窑精品。1975 年扬州市东风砖瓦厂出土。

扬州博物馆藏

This ewer has a trumpet mouth, a high neck, a sloping shoulder, a pie-shaped foot and a flat bottom with the lower part of its long, round belly tapering downwards. Connecting the neck to the shoulder is a composite loop handle, opposite which is a round short spout. Regularly refined, the base of the body is firm and fine, showing elegant shape. Engobe can be found between the body and the white glaze. This ewer is a fine example of porcelain produced in Xing kiln, Hebei Province. It was unearthed in Dongfeng brick kiln in Yangzhou, Jiangsu Province, in the year 1975.

Preserved in Yangzhou Museum

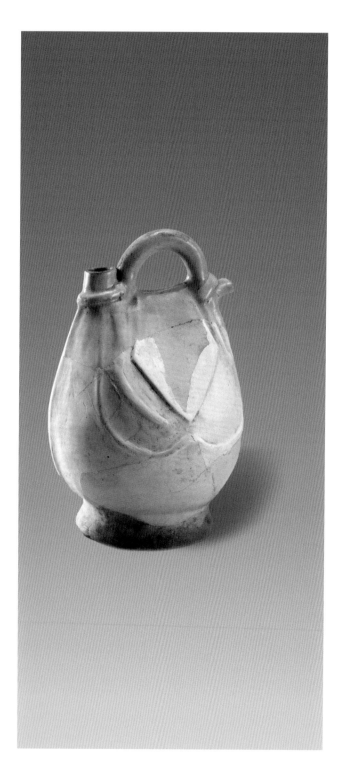

白釉皮囊形壶

唐

瓷质

最大腹径 15.6 厘米，底径 10.6 厘米，高 22.6
厘米

White-glazed Flask in the Shape of Leather Bag

Tang Dynasty

Porcelain

Maximum Belly Diameter 15.6 cm/ Bottom
Diameter 10.6 cm/ Height 22.6 cm

壶体呈上扁下鼓，似皮囊状。上左侧有一管状直流，流下有一圈凸起的单环；上右侧有一扁平翘起的尾状把手，上有圆弧状的提梁，圈足底。壶腹两侧采用堆贴并刻画弧形条状纹。白釉白胎，外釉不及底，釉下施化妆土。釉面较光润发亮，釉色白中微泛黄，有细裂纹开片。河南巩县窑烧制。1991 年扬州市区文昌阁东南侧唐代文化层中出土。

扬州博物馆藏

This flask with an oblate upper part and a bulging lower part looks like a leather bag. On the left side of its upper part is a straight tubiform spout, and below the spout is a single circle of convex hoop. On its right side is a flat handle resembling a cocked tail, while on its top is placed an arc loop handle. It has a ring foot. With the combination of embossed decoration, both sides of the flask are incised with arc-shaped strip lines. Its white body is covered with white glaze, except for the bottom, and engobe is painted under the glaze. The white shiny mellow glaze shows tints of yellow and tiny crackles. The flask was fired in the kiln of Gong County, Henan Province, and it was unearthed in 1991 from the culture layer of the Tang Dynasty on the south-east side of the Wenchang Pavilion in Yangzhou, Jiangsu Province.

Preserved in Yangzhou Museum

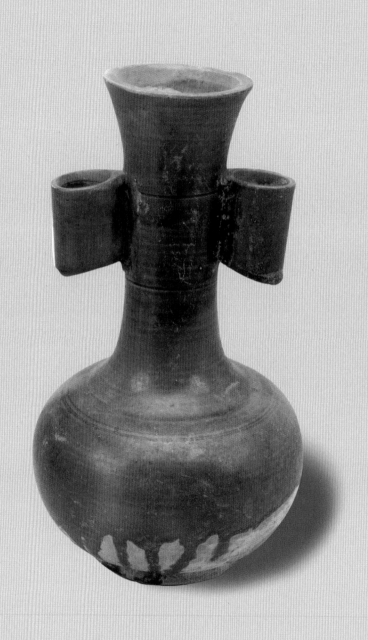

赭釉双耳投壶

唐

瓷质

高 35 厘米

喇叭口，长颈，颈两侧贴附筒形双耳，左右对称，溜肩，鼓腹，平底，圈足。投壶是古代宴会上的一种礼仪活动。

陕西省昭陵博物馆藏

Ochre-glazed Vase with Double Ears

Tang Dynasty

Porcelain

Height 35 cm

The vase is characterized with an inverted trumpet-shaped mouth, a long neck with cylindrical ears symmetrically attached at each side, a sloping shoulder, a drum belly, a flat bottom and a ring foot. The Chinese name of this kind of vase is Touhu, which was derived from an ancient game, and later became a ritual activity held at a banquet in ancient times.

Preserved in Zhaoling Museum, Shaanxi Province

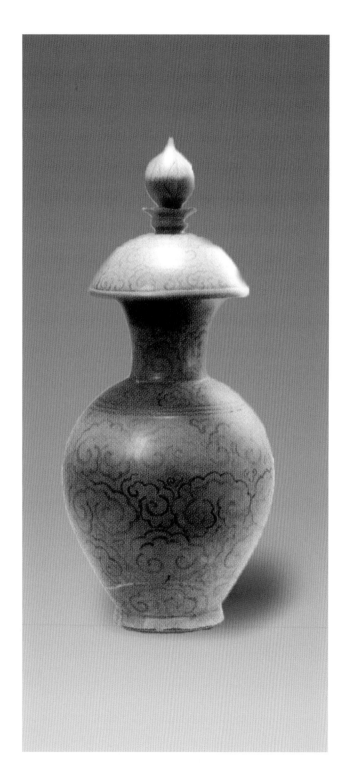

釉下彩绘瓷盖罂

唐

瓷质

口径 20 厘米，通高 64.5 厘米

Covered Small-mouthed Jar with Under-glazed Paints

Tang Dynasty

Porcelain

Mouth Diameter 20 cm/ Height 64.5 cm

盘口式颈，鼓腹平底，盘口之上另有覆钵式盖，盖的外廓线与罂肩腹曲线上下呼应，形成一个流畅的卵形。盖顶的把手做成圆形花蕾，使整个已封闭的卵形顿显修长挺拔，整体造型优雅，曲线柔美。通体施釉，青中泛黄。釉下为褐彩绘出的如意头形卷云纹。釉色与纹样搭配非常协调。浙江省临安区出土。

浙江省博物馆藏

This jar has a neck in the shape of a dish-mouth, a bulging belly and a flat bottom. Above the mouth is a cover, resembling a diverted bowl. The outlines of the cover and the curve of the shoulder and the belly of the jar, in concert with each other, form a smooth oval shape. The knob on its cover is shaped into a flower bud, making the enclosing oval slenderer and taller. Elegant in shape, the whole vessel presents a graceful figure. It is fully glazed cyan with a hint of yellow, and under the glaze are Ruyi-shaped cloud patterns painted in brown colour. The glaze colour matches well with the decorative patterns. The jar was unearthed from Lin'an District, Zhejiang Province.

Preserved in Zhejiang Museum

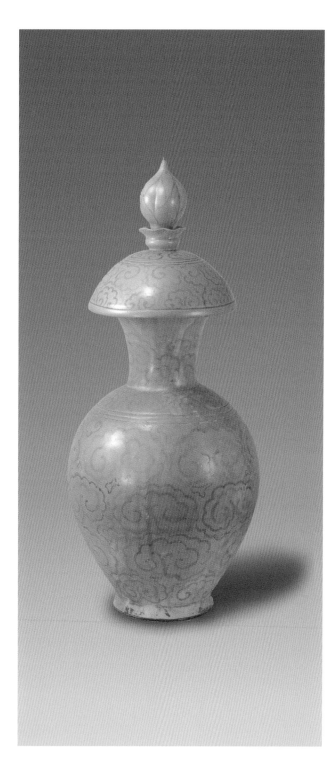

褐彩如意云纹青瓷罂

唐

瓷质

口径 19.8 厘米，底径 16 厘米，高 66.5 厘米

Small-Mouthed Celadon Jar with Brown "Ruyi" Pattern

Tang Dynasty

Porcelain

Mouth Diameter 19.8 cm/ Bottom Diameter 16 cm/

Height 66.5 cm

盖上制成含苞欲放的莲花。通体青釉呈青黄色。包括盖面在内通体均绘釉下褐彩如意云纹。此件罂与同墓出土的熏炉高度相仿，大型器物制作如此精美，实属罕见，可谓晚唐越窑青瓷之佳作。1980 年临安区唐水邱氏墓出土。

临安市文物馆藏

The knob on the lid is shaped into a lotus in bud. The whole vessel is coated with green glaze with a greenish-yellow shine, and is decorated with brown underglazed Ruyi patterns. It is similar in height to the censer unearthed from the same tomb. This exquisite large-sized vessel is a masterpiece produced by Yue kiln in the late Tang dynasty. It was unearthed from the Shuiqiu family tomb of the Tang Dynasty in Lin'an District, Zhejiang Province, in the year 1980.

Preserved in Lin'an Museum of Cultural Relics

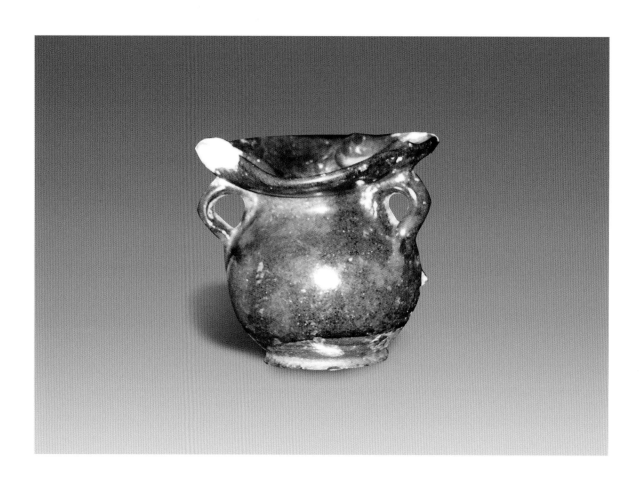

黑釉双耳盂

唐

瓷质

口径 8 厘米，底径 4 厘米，通高 7 厘米，重 150 克

Black-glazed Spittoon with Two Ears

Tang Dynasty

Porcelain

Mouth Diameter 8 cm/ Bottom Diameter 4 cm/ Height 7 cm/ Weight 150 g

盘口，圆腹，平底，口有三凸棱，双耳，下腹
无釉。生活用器。口有修补。

陕西医史博物馆藏

The spittoon, with a plate-shaped mouth, a
round belly and a flat bottom, is an object for
daily use. Under the mouth are two ears with
three ridge lines. The lower part of the belly is
unglazed. The mouth has been restored.

Preserved in Shaanxi Museum of Medical History

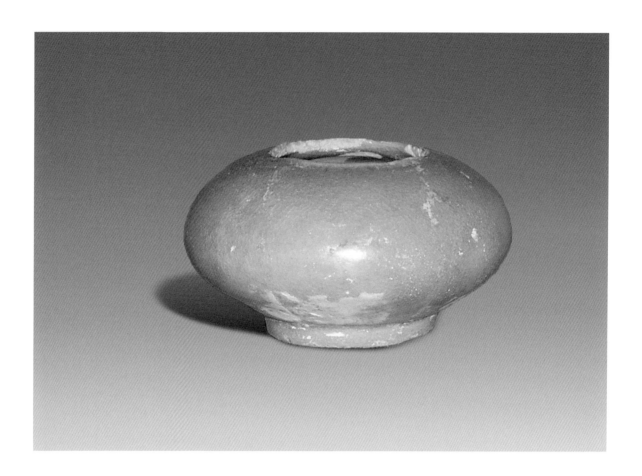

瓷盂

唐

瓷质

口径 3 厘米，底径 3.5 厘米，通高 38 厘米，重 100 克

Porcelain Water Pot

Tang Dynasty

Porcelain

Mouth Diameter 3 cm/ Bottom Diameter3.5 cm/ Height 38 cm/ Weight 100 g

弇口，鼓腹，平底，黄瓷。生活用器。有裂印。

陕西省西安市何家村征集。

陕西医史博物馆藏

The yellow water pot, with a small mouth, a swelling belly, and a flat bottom, is a household utensil. The pot was cracked, and it was collected in Hejia Village, Xi'an, Shaanxi Province.

Preserved in Shaanxi Museum of Medical History

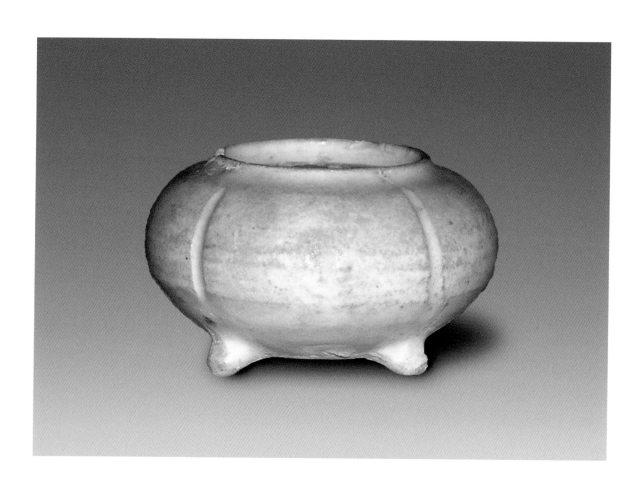

三足盂

唐

瓷质

口径 4.5 厘米，底径 3.8 厘米，通高 3.7 厘米，重 100 克

Water Pot with Tripod Foot

Tang Dynasty

Porcelain

Mouth Diameter 4.5 cm/ Bottom Diameter 3.8 cm/ Height 3.7 cm/ Weight 100 g

弇口，鼓腹，三乳丁足，腹有等距四条竖纹，

白瓷。生活用器。口沿有缺。陕西省西安市

何家村征集。

陕西医史博物馆藏

This pot has a small mouth, whose rim was damaged, a swelling belly decorated with four equidistant vertical stripes, and a tripod foot. It was a household vessel, collected in Hejia Village, Xi'an, Shaanxi Province.

Preserved in Shaanxi Museum of Medical History

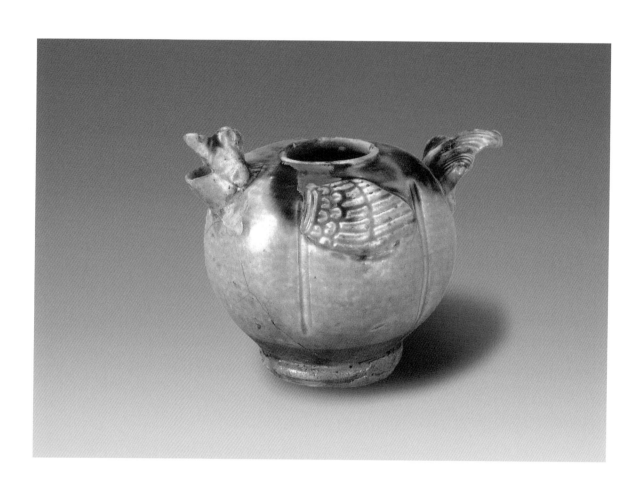

青釉褐绿彩鸟形水注

唐

瓷质

口径 3 厘米，腹径 8.7 厘米，底径 5 厘米，高 9 厘米

Celadon Bird-shaped Water Pot with Tints of Brownish Green

Tang Dynasty

Porcelain

Mouth Diameter 3 cm/ Belly Diameter 8.7 cm/ Bottom Diameter 5 cm/ Height 9 cm

整个器形呈瓜楞鸟首状，平口，口沿微出，饼足底，口沿、上腹施绿褐彩，鼓腹，腹部分四条直棱成瓜棱状。鸟首张开形成注流，鸟尾自然伸展，成为把手。腹部上端两侧堆贴，刻画成鸟翅，造型生动，形象逼真。青黄色釉，釉面光洁，外釉不及底。1995年扬州市区皇宫唐代灰坑中出土。

扬州博物馆藏

This water pot, in the shape of a melon with a bird head, has a flat mouth, with the rim slightly protruding outwards, and a pie-shaped foot. Its melon-shaped belly has four straight concave lines, like those on a pumpkin. Its mouth rim and upper belly are coated with brownish-green glaze. The mouth of the bird acts as the spout of the pot, while the tail extends naturally into the handle. The two sides of the upper belly are incised with vivid bird's wings. The vessel is covered with lustrous and smooth greenish-yellow glaze, while the base is left unglazed. It was unearthed in an imperial pit of the Tang Dynasty in Yangzhou, Jiangsu Province, in 1995.

Preserved in Yangzhou Museum

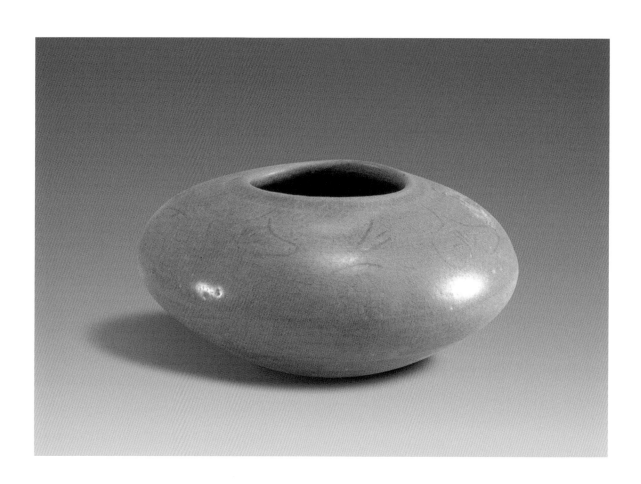

水盂

唐

瓷质

口径 3.8 厘米，高 4.4 厘米

Water Pot

Tang Dynasty

Porcelain

Mouth Diameter 3.8 cm/ Height 4.4 cm

敛口，鼓腹，下腹内收甚，小平底略上凹。上
腹刻画荷叶纹，施青釉，外底无釉。

浙江省文物考古研究所藏

This pot has a contracted mouth, a swelling
belly, whose lower part tapers down sharply. Its
small flat bottom is slightly concaved-upward.
The upper belly is covered with celadon glaze,
and engraved with lotus leaf patterns. The outer
bottom is unglazed.

Preserved in Institute of Cultural Relics and
Archaeology of Zhejiang Province

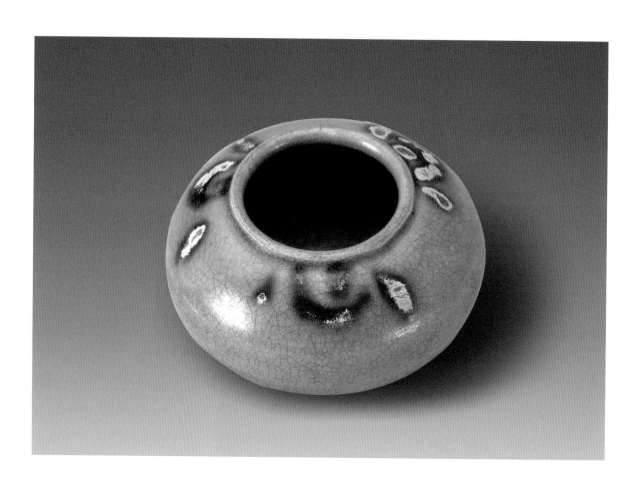

青釉绿彩"心"字水盂

唐

瓷质

口径 4.1 厘米，底径 3.7 厘米，高 4.3 厘米

Celadon-glazed Water Pot with Green-glazed Chinese Character "Xin"

Tang Dynasty

Porcelain

Mouth Diameter 4.1 cm/ Bottom Diameter 3.7 cm/ Height 4.3 cm

其造型精致小巧，敛口光沿，溜肩鼓腹，饼形
足。器表满施青釉，釉面开冰裂纹，沿口外侧
有绿彩间隔书写三个"心"字，用笔率意，布
局合理，"三心"紧贴口沿自然天成，趣味横
生。此件水盂具有典型的长沙窑工艺特征，在
目前所发现的长沙窑小水盂中应为妙品。1996
年扬州市开发区工地出土。

扬州博物馆藏

This pot, exquisitely designed, has a contracted
mouth with a smooth rim, a sloping shoulder, a
convex belly and a pie-shaped foot. The exterior
of the pot is coated with celadon glaze with
ice crackles. On the outside wall, below the
mouth rim is a green-glazed Chinese character
"Xin" written in three directions in a simple
natural style. The three "Xin" characters are
placed naturally along the mouth rim. The pot
exemplifies typical porcelain ware produced in
Changsha kiln, and is a masterpiece of the small
water pots made in that area. It was unearthed
in a construction site of the Development Zone
in Yangzhou, Jiangsu Province, in 1996.
Preserved in Yangzhou Museum

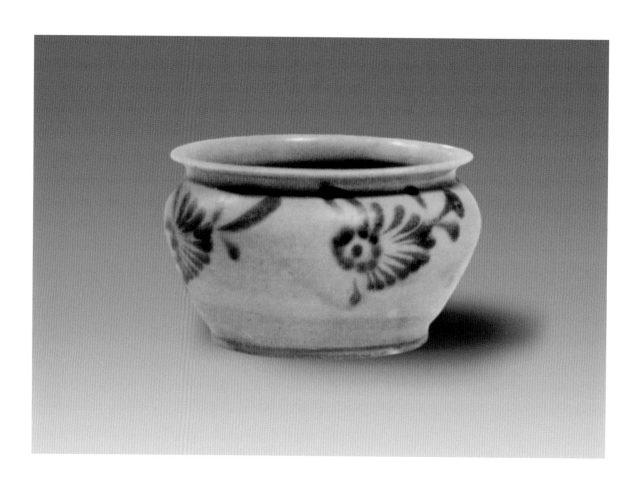

釉下彩绘瓷水盂

唐

瓷质

口径 16 厘米，高 9.7 厘米

Under-glazed Water Pot

Tang Dynasty

Porcelain

Mouth Diameter 16 cm/ Height 9.7 cm

大口矮领，硕腹平底。胎体呈褐红色，胎上罩一层白色为底，既掩盖了胎面上的瑕疵，又增强了彩绘母题的效果，这便是瓷器中惯常使用的化妆土技法。在化妆土上，以含铁、铜成分的颜料勾画出几组极似飞鸟的蔓草，然后于整个器表施一层青黄色彩。这便是著名的唐代长沙窑釉下彩绘瓷器。湖南省长沙县出土。

长沙博物馆藏

This pot has a big mouth, a short neck, a large belly and a flat bottom. On its brownish red body is a layer of white engobe, which not only covers the body's flaws, but also reinforces the effect of painted motif. It is a commonly used engobe technique in porcelain production. On the top of the engobe are painted several bird-like trailing plants patterns with colourants containing iron and copper, while the outermost exterior is coated with bluish-yellow glaze. This pot exemplifies the famous under-glaze porcelain made in Changsha kiln in the Tang Dynasty. It was unearthed in Changsha County, Hunan Province.

Preserved in Changsha Museum

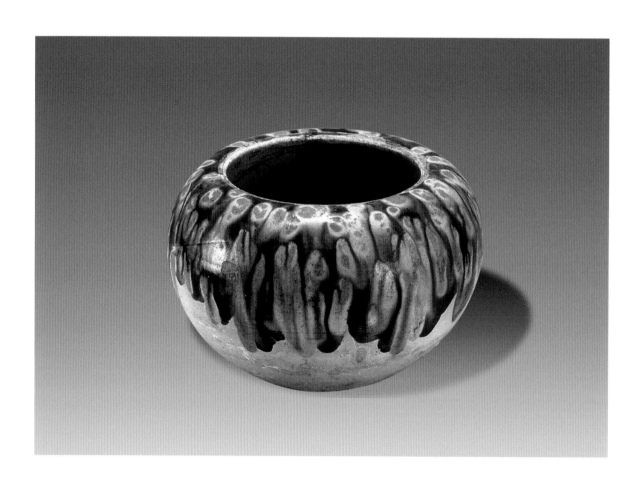

三彩钵盂

唐

瓷质

口径 13.5 厘米，高 14.5 厘米

Tricolour Alms Bowl

Tang Dynasty

Porcelain

Mouth Diameter 13.5 cm/ Height 14.5 cm

钵盂口内敛，肩稍耸，鼓腹，小平底。外腹施黄、绿、白、褐四色釉，釉面斑驳交融，绚丽自然。垂釉不及底，露白胎，胎质细腻，胎体厚重。该器形敦实沉稳，极其实用。1958 年扬州市五台山出土。

扬州博物馆藏

The alms bowl has a contracted mouth, a slightly shrugged shoulder, a swelling belly and a small flat bottom. The outside of its belly is coated with gracefully and naturally mixed glazes in yellow, green, white and brown. The lower part and the bottom are left unglazed, exposing its white thick body, fine and smooth in texture. This type of ware looks stocky and is extremely practical. It was unearthed from Mount Wutai, Yangzhou, Jiangsu Province, in the year 1958.
Preserved in Yangzhou Museum

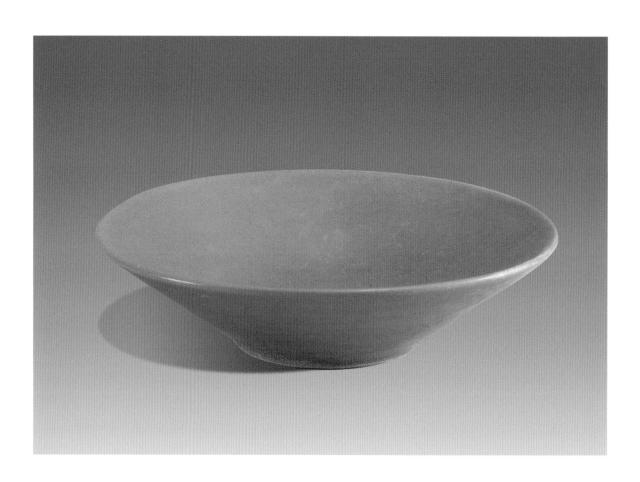

碗

唐

瓷质

口径 14.2 厘米，高 3.8 厘米

Bowl

Tang Dynasty

Porcelain

Mouth Diameter 14.2 cm/ Height 3.8 cm

敞口，斜直腹，玉璧形足。满青釉，足底外缘刮釉。1994 年慈溪市上林湖荷花蕊窑址出土。

浙江省文物考古研究所藏

This bowl has a wide mouth, a straight body tapering to a jade-disk-shaped bottom. The interior and exterior of the bowl are fully coated with celadon glaze. The glaze on the outer edge of the bottom is scraped off. It was unearthed in the Hehuarui kiln ruins in Shanglinhu, Cixi, Zhengjiang Province, in the year 1994.

Preserved in Institute of Cultural Relics and Archaeology of Zhejiang Province

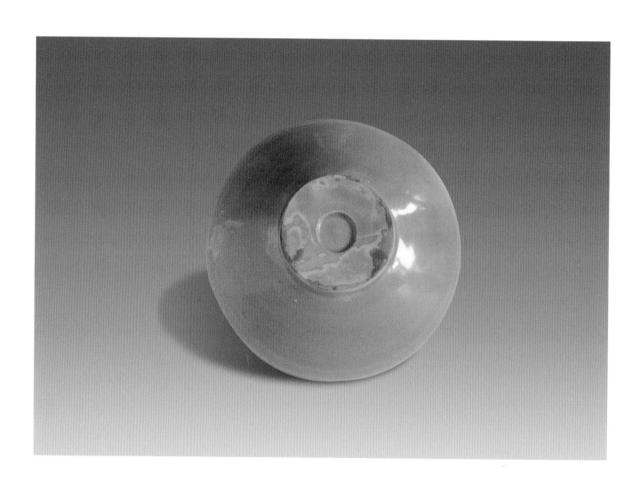

越窑青釉碗

唐

瓷质

口径 13 厘米

Celadon-glazed Bowl, Yue Ware

Tang Dynasty

Porcelain

Mouth Diameter 13 cm

敞口，浅腹，玉璧足，施青绿色釉至足部，足脐内亦有釉，可见三垫烧痕，灰白胎，甚坚细，釉面有土侵痕迹。越窑是唐、五代、北宋初著名瓷窑，以浙江上虞窑寺前、帐子山、凌湖、余姚上林湖等产地为代表。初唐越窑器物仍处在中国青瓷低潮时期，中唐以后质量逐渐提高，有"类玉""类冰"及"千峰翠色"之誉。唐人陆羽《茶经》评价青瓷茶盏，置越窑于第一。其较好的产品称"秘色瓷"。

黄卓文藏

This bowl has a wide mouth, a shallow belly and a jade-disk-shaped bottom. It is coated with green glaze thoroughly which runs even to the bottom umbilicus. There are three pad-like firing marks on the bottom. Its greyish-white body is of extremely firm and fine texture. Its surface shows traces of clay contamination. Yue kiln was well-known in the Tang Dynasty, the Five Dynasties, and the early Northern Song Dynasty, and was represented by kilns in Zhejiang Province, such as Yaosiqian in Shangyu, Mount Zhangzi, Ling Lake and Shanglin Lake in Yuyao. In the early Tang Dynasty, celadon porcelain ware made in Yue kiln was not well known yet, while after the middle Tang dynasty, the quality of Yue ware was improved gradually, winning such complimentary comments as "jade-like", "ice-like", and "like the green colour of a thousand mountain summits". Lu Yu, a famous figure in the Tang Dynasty wrote in *The Book of Tea* that Yue ware was the best celadon-glazed tea ware. High quality Yue ware is called "secret colour porcelain".
Collected by Huang Zhuowen

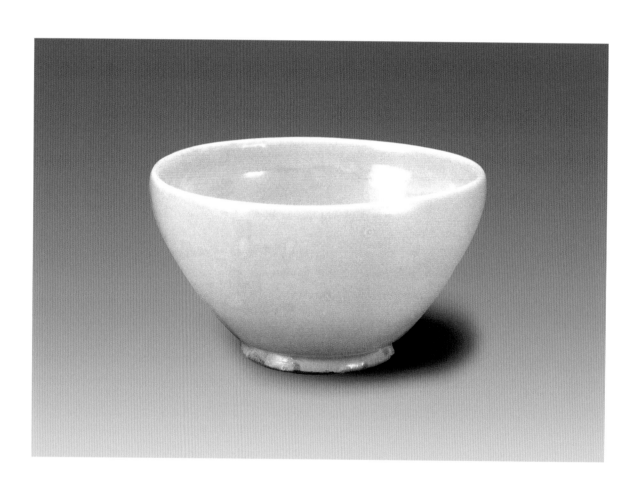

白釉碗

唐

瓷质

底长 9.1 厘米，底宽 8 厘米，高 11.5 厘米

White-glazed Bowl

Tang Dynasty

Porcelain

Base Length 9.1 cm/ Base Width 8 cm/ Height 11.5 cm

白釉碗产于唐代北方的邢窑。邢窑尤以出产碗壶居多。碗敛口，碗壁至足稍带弧度呈喇叭状，圈足聚釉处略呈水绿色，圈足偶露胎色。白釉碗胎骨坚实致密，胎色洁白，修坯规整，瓷化程度高，其釉面滋润，有白玉感。正如唐代陆羽《茶经》中所述"白如雪，类似银"。1992 年扬州四望亭南段怡园工地采集。

扬州博物馆藏

This white-glazed bowl was made in the Tang Dynasty in Xing kiln, a kiln in the north of China, in which lots of bowls and pots were produced. The bowl, with a contracted mouth, is shaped into a trumpet with a slight radian shown from the wall to the foot. The ring foot, where the glaze gathers, is in aqua, while the unglazed part of the foot exposes the white body. The texture of its body is firm and dense, and the colour is purely white. The fettling is regularly made and it is highly vitrified with mellow lustrous glaze resembling white jade, just like what was remarked by Lu Yu, a famous figure in the Tang Dynasty in *The Book Of Tea*: "as white as snow, and similar to silver". It was collected in the year 1992 from Yiyuan construction site in the south section of Siwang Pavilion, Yangzhou, Jiangsu Province.

Preserved in Yangzhou Museum

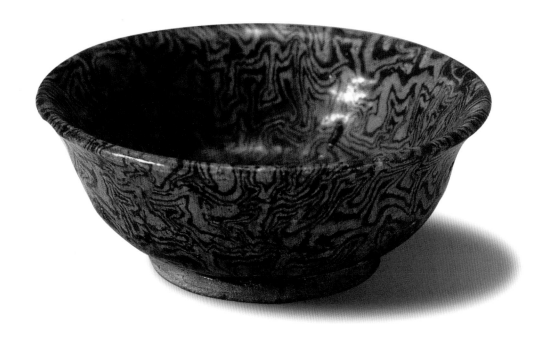

黄釉搅胎碗

唐

瓷质

口径 10.4 厘米，底径 5.4 厘米，高 4.2 厘米

Yellow-glazed Bowl with Twisted Clay

Tang Dynasty

Porcelain

Mouth Diameter 10.4 cm/ Bottom Diameter 5.4 cm/ Height 4.2 cm

敞口外撇，圈足底。此碗是用褐色和白色两种
颜色瓷土相间糅合，经过拉坯成型，施淡黄釉
焙烧而成。唯圈足胎色单一。此碗纹理变化多
端，犹如行云流水。搅胎是唐代陶瓷业中的一
种新工艺，为河南巩县窑产品。1990 年扬州
市汶河北路信托大厦工地出土。

扬州博物馆藏

This bowl made with twisted clay has a wide
flared mouth and a ring foot. The bowl is of
brown and white clay, and is produced through
the process of casting, glazing and firing. Only
the ring foot presents a single colour. The
bowl's texture is tortuous and irregular, like
floating clouds and flowing water. Twisted clay
was invented by the kiln of Gong County in
Henan Province in the Tang Dynasty. It was
unearthed from the construction site of Trust
Building on Wenhe North Road in Yangzhou,
Jiangsu Province, in the year 1990.

Preserved in Yangzhou Museum

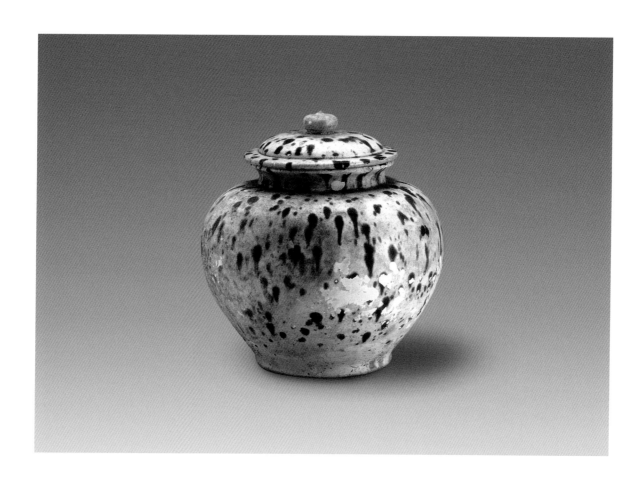

白釉蓝彩盖罐

唐

瓷质

口径 10.4 厘米，通高 17.8 厘米

Covered White-glazed Jar with Blue Spots

Tang Dynasty

Porcelain

Mouth Diameter 10.4 cm/ Height 17.8 cm

侈口，束颈，鼓腹，下腹渐收，平底。上置扁平盖，扁圆钮。胎白且细腻。满施白釉，色微泛黄，通体以蓝釉洒点成自然的纹饰，如潇潇雨下，颇具特色。1974 年扬州市城北乡红星村出土。

扬州博物馆藏

This jar has a wide flared mouth, a contracted neck, a bulging belly, the lower part of which tapers down gradually, and a flat bottom. It has a flat lid with an oblate knob. The fine white body is covered with white glaze with a tint of yellow. The whole jar is decorated with blue-glazed speckles in the form of rain drops. It was unearthed in Hongxing Village, Chengbei Township, Yangzhou, Jiangsu Province, in 1974.

Preserved in Yangzhou Museum

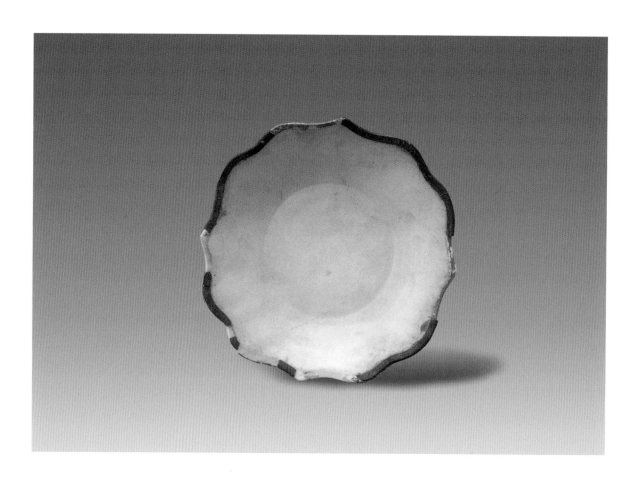

白瓷花口盘

唐

瓷质

口径 15 厘米，底径 6 厘米，高 3 厘米

White Porcelain Plate with Flower-petal-shaped Mouth

Tang Dynasty

Porcelain

Mouth Diameter 15 cm/ Bottom Diameter 6 cm/ Height 3 cm

胎壁极薄，有半透明之感，口沿和圈足镶金银

扣，外底刻"新官"款。

临安市文物馆藏

The body of this plate is so thin that it is almost
translucent, and the mouth rim and the foot ring
are bound with silver and gold. The outside
bottom is incised with two Chinese characters
"Xin Guan".
Preserved in Lin'an Museum of Cultural Relics

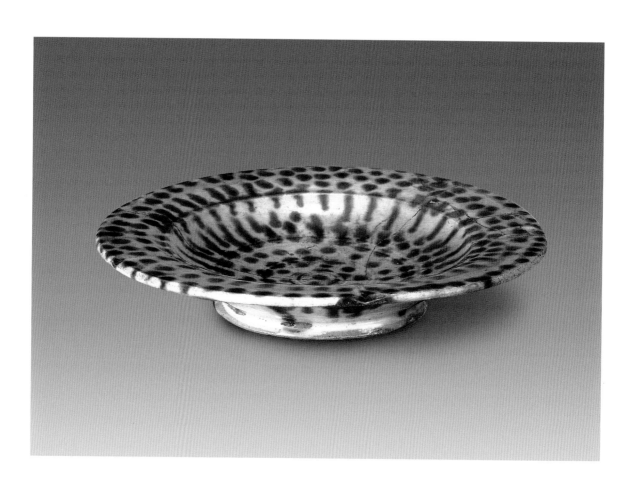

白釉点绿彩盘

唐

瓷质

口径 25.6 厘米，底径 12.4 厘米，高 4.8 厘米

White-glazed Plate with Green Speckles

Tang Dynasty

Porcelain

Mouth Diameter 25.6 cm/ Bottom Diameter 12.4 cm/ Height 4.8 cm

平口宽沿，折腹，圈足底。外壁点绿彩斑块，内壁点连珠绿彩，点彩疏密有致。白釉，红褐色胎，胎质较细密，釉面光洁发亮，华丽典雅。从胎质釉色来看，与扬州唐代遗址出土的一批唐代白釉绿彩瓷一致，为河南巩县窑烧制。1991年扬州市区文昌阁东南侧唐代文化层出土。

扬州博物馆藏

This plate has a flat mouth with a wide rim, an angular belly, and a ring foot. On the exterior and interior walls are green-glazed speckles. The speckles on the interior wall resemble chains of pearls arranged in a reasonable layout. With its fine reddish-brown body covered with smooth and luminous white glaze, the plate looks beautiful and elegant. Judged from its body texture and glaze colour, it is in accord with the white-glazed porcelains with green speckles of the Tang Dynasty, unearthed from the ruins of the Tang Dynasty in Yangzhou, Jiangsu Province, and all of them were made in the kiln of Gong County in Henan Province. It was unearthed from the culture layer of the Tang Dynasty on the south-east side of the Wenchang Pavilion in Yangzhou, Jiangsu Province, in 1991.

Preserved in Yangzhou Museum

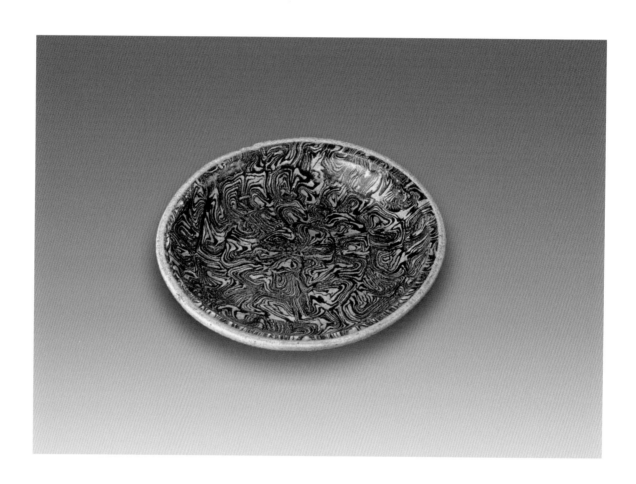

绞胎纹瓷盘

唐

瓷质

口径 17.1 厘米，底径 11.8 厘米，高 2.1 厘米

Plate with Twisted Clay

Tang Dynasty

Porcelain

Mouth Diameter 17.1 cm/ Bottom Diameter 11.8 cm/ Height 2.1 cm

平沿方唇，浅腹平底，胎体厚重，盘内外满布类似木质纹理样的几何图案，且内外完全一致。这就是唐代新出现的陶瓷装饰工艺 = 绞胎（或称搅胎或搅泥，是一种借鉴漆器装饰美化陶瓷的技法）。盛食器皿。

山东博物院藏

This plate has a flat mouth, a square-shaped rim, a shallow belly, a flat bottom and a thick body. The interior and exterior of the plate are decorated with geometric patterns in wood-like texture. Twisted clay techniques were new porcelain decoration techniques invented in the Tang Dynasty, which were derived from and inspired by the lacquerwork technique. The plate used to serve food.

Preserved in Shandong Museum

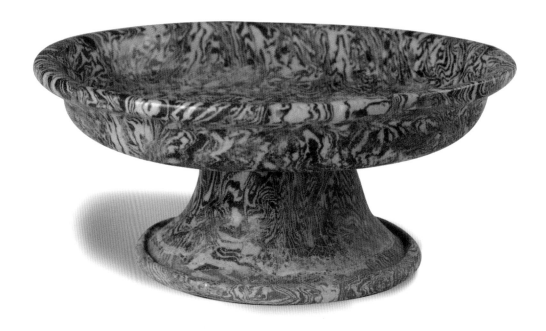

绞胎高足盘

唐

瓷质

口径 13.2 厘米，底径 7.8 厘米，高 5.3 厘米

High-Stemmed Plate with Twisted Clay

Tang Dynasty

Porcelain

Mouth Diameter 13.2 cm/ Bottom Diameter 7.8 cm/ Height 5.3 cm

口撇卷唇，浅腹，中空的高足似喇叭状。足近底处向上卷起成一凸弦纹。盘内、外满釉，釉莹润透亮，开细纹片。近脚处与内底无釉，胎露白，褐色两色相间，所以称为绞胎。绞胎作品盛于唐、五代，该盘是晚唐代表作品。

林炽基藏

This plate has a flared mouth with a rolled rim, a shallow belly and a tall, hollow and trumpet-shaped foot. The portion close to the bottom rolls upward forming a string pattern. Both the interior and exterior of the plate are coated with crackled glaze, which is bright, smooth and lustrous, while the portion near the bottom and the interior of the bottom are unglazed, exposing the body which is mingled by brown and white clay, also called twisted clay. Porcelain vessels with twisted clay flourished in the Tang dynasty and the Five Dynasties. This plate is a masterpiece of the Late Tang Dynasty.

Collected by Li Chiji

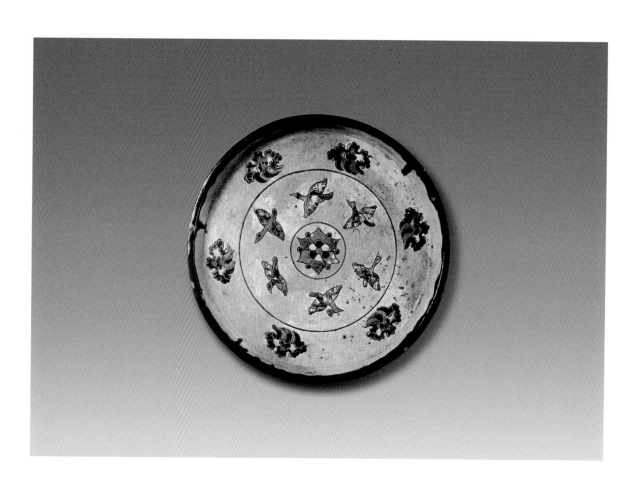

三彩飞鸟云纹盘

唐

瓷质

口径 31.6 厘米，高 6.4 厘米

Tricolour Plate with Bird and Cloud Patterns

Tang Dynasty

Porcelain

Mouth Diameter 31.6 cm/ Height 6.4 cm

厚厚的方唇，短短的立壁和宽敞的平底，颇有
唐人气度。绳索状环形矮足既随意又极具装饰
意味。盘内图案的布局与色调甚为考究，无论
是中心花朵黄绿相间、黑白相次的用色，还是
飞鸟与流云的对应构图，都给人以严谨工整的
感觉。口沿部位墨绿的釉色在浅黄地的衬托下
充满了勃勃生机。

上海博物馆藏

With a thick square-shaped lip, a short vertical
wall and a wide flat bottom, this plate bears
the styles and characteristics of the people
in the Tang Dynasty. The randomly arranged
rope-shaped short ring foot serves well as
a decoration. The layout and colours of the
patterns in the plate are carefully designed.
Both the colours of the central flowers, either
in yellow and green, or in black and white, and
the design of flying birds corresponding with
floating clouds convey the sense of preciseness
and order. The dark green glaze on the
mouth rim looks vigorous on the light yellow
background.

Preserved in Shanghai Museum

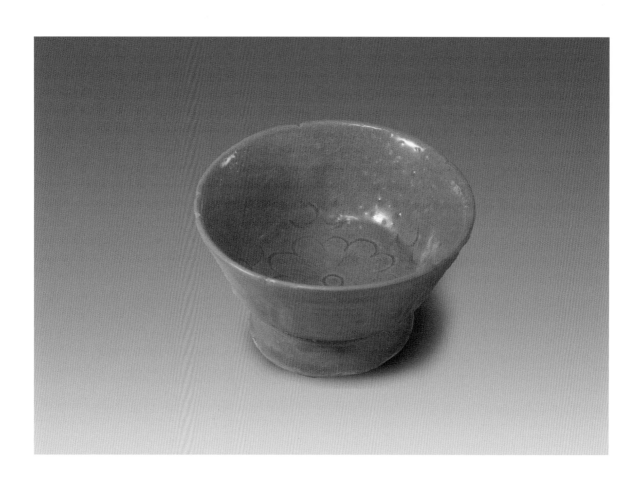

盏

唐

瓷质

口径 12 厘米，高 7 厘米

Cup

Tang Dynasty

Porcelain

Mouth Diameter 12 cm/ Height 7 cm

敞口，腹斜直，圈足外撇较高。口有五个凹
缺，外腹压出五道短痕，使整器呈荷花状。内
底刻画荷叶纹，满青釉，足底有 10 个泥点痕。
1994 年慈溪市上林湖荷花蕊窑址出土。

浙江省文物考古研究所藏

The cup has a flared mouth, a steep-sided belly,
and a stem flared ring foot. With five-lobed
mouth rim and five concave lines along the
exterior of the belly, the cup looks like a lotus.
The inside of the bottom is incised with lotus
patterns while the outside has ten clay speckle
marks. The cup is coated with celadon glaze.
It was unearthed from the Hehuarui kiln ruin
in Shanglinhu, Cixi, Zhejiang Province, in the
year 1994.
Preserved in Institute of Cultural Relics and
Archaeology of Zhejiang Province

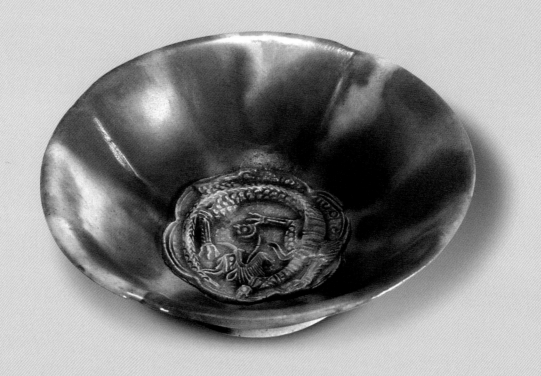

绿釉模印堆塑龙纹盏

唐

瓷质

口径 14.6 厘米，底径 6.9 厘米，高 4.3 厘米

Green-glazed Cup with a Moulded Dragon

Tang Dynasty

Porcelain

Mouth Diameter 14.6 cm/ Bottom Diameter 6.9 cm/ Height 4.3 cm

盏为四瓣葵形，口沿外侈，斜弧腹，圈足外撇。外腹及足心各有两道凹弦纹。盏心堆塑一条蟠龙。龙尖嘴，身披鳞甲，四爪伸开，张口吐珠，短尾盘于腹下。龙身四周饰云气纹。河南巩县窑烧制的不可多得的艺术精品。1983 年于扬州市三元路出土。

扬州博物馆藏

With a flared mouth, a sloping belly, and a flared ring foot, this cup is in the shape of a sunflower with four petals. There are two incised lines on the exterior belly and the centre of the base, respectively. At the centre of the cup is moulded a curled-up dragon among the cloud. The dragon coated with scales has a sharp speak, four claws stretching out, a pearl in the mouth, and a short tail under the belly. The cup is a masterpiece made in the kiln of Gong County in Henan Province. It was unearthed from Sanyuan Road, Yangzhou, Jiangsu Province, in 1983.

Preserved in Yangzhou Museum

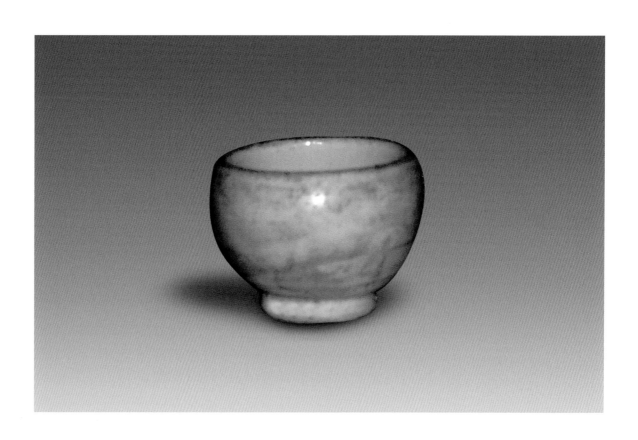

小酒杯

唐

瓷质

口径 3.5 厘米，底径 2 厘米，通高 2.6 厘米，重
1750 克

敛口，圆腹，圈足，白瓷。酒器。完整无损。陕
西省西安市征集。

陕西医史博物馆藏

Tass

Tang Dynasty

Porcelain

Mouth Diameter 3.5 cm/ Bottom Diameter 2 cm/
Height 2.6 cm/ Weight 1,750 g

This tass, a small wine cup, is characterized with
a contracted mouth, a round belly, and a ring foot.
It has been kept intact. It was collected in Xi'an,
Shaanxi Province.

Preserved in Shaanxi Museum of Medical History

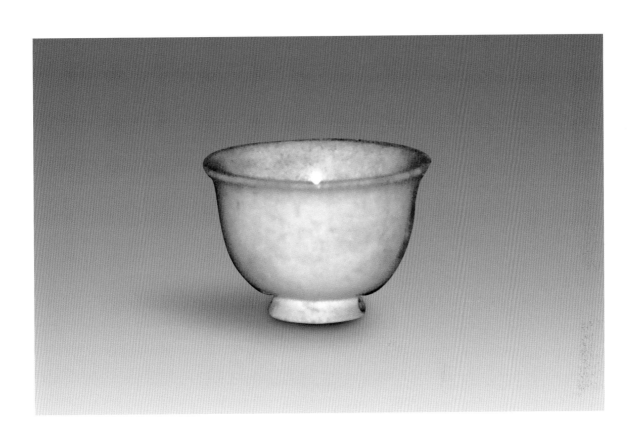

小酒杯

唐

瓷质

口径 3.4 厘米，底径 0.9 厘米，通高 2.2 厘米，重
1050 克

敞口，圆腹，圈足，白瓷。酒器。完整无损。陕
西省西安市征集。

陕西医史博物馆藏

Tass

Tang Dynasty

White porcelain

Mouth Diameter 3.4 cm/ Bottom Diameter 0.9 cm/
Height 2.2 cm/ Weight 1,050 g

This tass, a wine cup, has a flared mouth, a round
belly and a ring foot. It has been kept intact. It was
collected in Xi'an, Shaanxi Province.

Preserved in Shaanxi Museum of Medical History

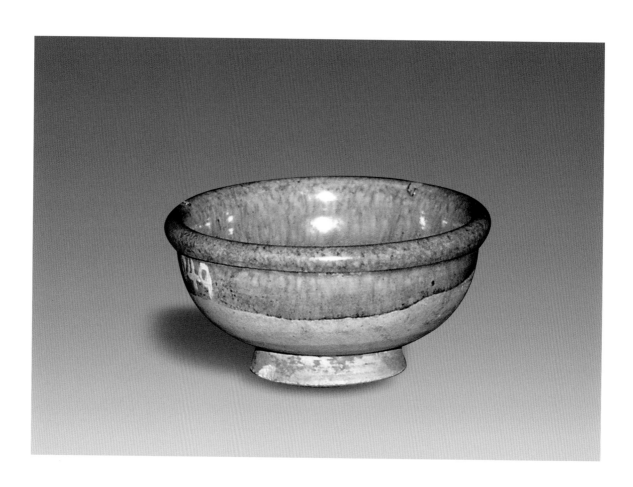

黄釉杯

唐

瓷质

口径 6.5 厘米，底径 3.1 厘米，通高 3.4 厘米，重 50 克

Yellow-glazed Cup

Tang Dynasty

Porcelain

Mouth Diameter 6.5 cm/ Bottom Diameter 3.1 cm/ Height 3.4 cm/ Weight 50 g

敞口，圆腹，碗内及口沿处黄釉，下腹白胎，

平底。生活用器。完整无损。陕西省西安市征集。

陕西医史博物馆藏

This cup has a flared mouth, a round belly and
a flat base. The interior wall and the mouth rim
are coated with yellow glaze, while the lower
belly and the foot are unglazed, exposing the
white body. The cup, a household utensil, is
perfectly preserved. It was collected in Xi'an,
Shaanxi Province.

Preserved in Shaanxi Museum of Medical History

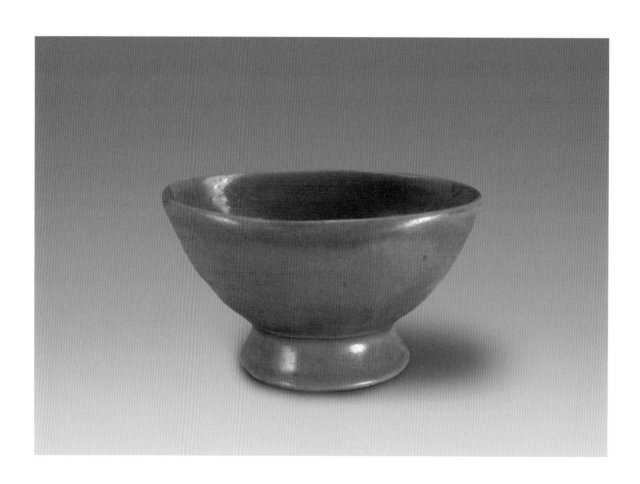

青釉船形杯

唐

瓷质

口长 11.6 厘米，口宽 7.8 厘米，底径 6.2 厘米，高 6.2 厘米

Celadon-glazed Cup in the Shape of a Boat

Tang Dynasty

Porcelain

Mouth Length 11.6 cm/ Mouth Width 7.8 cm/ Bottom Diameter 6.2 cm/ Height 6.2 cm

杯身呈船形，口沿略内敛，圈足底，足底圈有铁锈斑，足底部轮旋痕较明显。施满釉，釉色青中泛绿，釉面均匀光润，为越窑制品。1999 年扬州市区院大街南侧唐代排水沟中出土。

扬州博物馆藏

The cup has a boat-shaped body, a slightly contracted mouth and a ring foot. On the bottom of the foot are rust speckles and obvious wheel-shaped marks. The whole cup is coated with celadon glaze with a hint of green. Its glaze is smooth and mellow. It was made in Yue kiln, and was unearthed from a drainage canal of the Tang Dynasty on the south side of the Yuan Road in Yangzhou, Jiangsu Province, in the year 1999.

Preserved in Yangzhou Museum

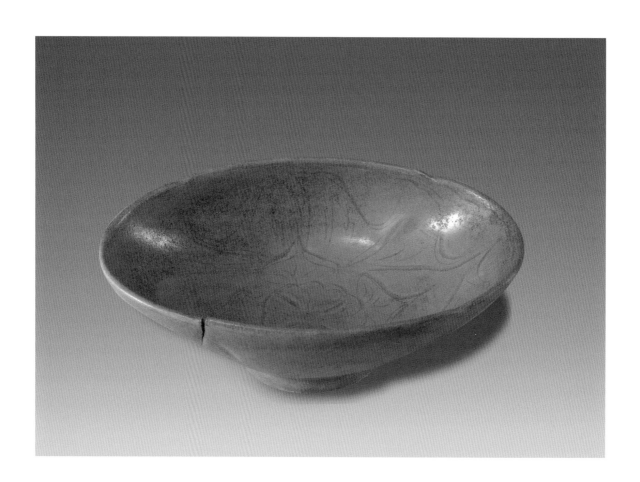

杯

唐

瓷质

长 14 厘米，宽 8.4 厘米，高 4.5 厘米

Cup

Tang Dynasty

Porcelain

Height 14 cm/ Width 8.4 cm/ Depth 4.5 cm

整器俯视呈椭圆形，口沿有相对的四个缺口，

缺下外腹压有四道短痕，内腹底刻画有荷叶纹，

满青釉，足底刮釉。1994 年慈溪市上林湖荷

花蕊窑址出土。

浙江省文物考古研究所藏

Seen from the top, the cup is in the shape
of an oval. On the mouth rim is incised four
symmetrical cuts from which four short curves
are stretched on the exterior stomach, and on
the interior bottom are carved lotus petals. The
cup is covered with rich green glaze, except the
foot rim. It was unearthed from Lianhuarui kiln
site by Shanglin Lake of Cixi City, Zhejiang
Province, in 1994.

Preserved in Institute of Cultural Relics and
Archaeology of Zhejiang Province

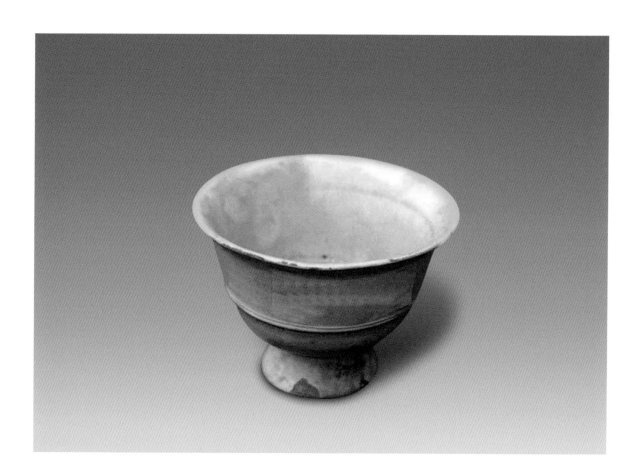

白釉高圈足杯

唐

瓷质

外口径 11.8 厘米，底径 5.7 厘米，通高 9 厘米，腹深 4.7 厘米，重 290 克

White-glazed Cup with High Stem

Tang Dynasty

Porcelain

Outer Mouth Diameter 11.8 cm/ Bottom Diameter 5.7 cm/ Height 9 cm/ Depth 4.7 cm/ Weight 290 g

敞口，圈足，杯身有两圈弦纹，盛饮料的器皿。

广东中医药博物馆藏

The cup has a flared mouth and a ring foot with two rings around the body. It was used as a wine vessel.

Preserved in Guangdong Chinese Medicine Museum

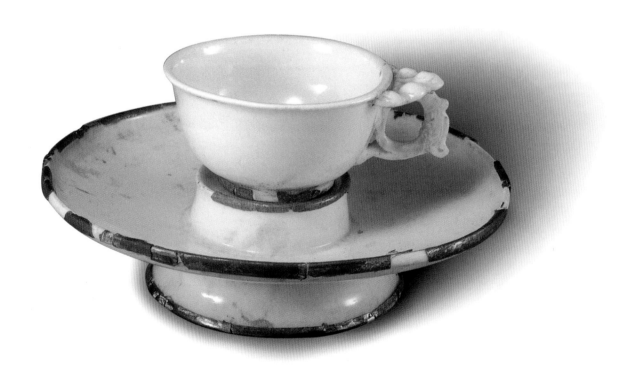

白瓷连托把杯

唐

瓷质

把杯：口径 8 厘米，高 4 厘米

托：高 4 厘米

杯一侧有如意形压手和圆环形柄，柄上浮雕一面为龙纹，一面作凤纹，寓意龙凤呈祥。刻纹精细流畅，釉色洁白滋润，颇具半透明感。圈足上包镶金银扣，底刻"新官"款。杯托之盘口、托沿、圈足均镶银扣，底刻"新官"款。

临安市文物馆藏

White Handled Cup with Saucer

Tang Dynasty

Porcelain

Handle Cup: Mouth Diameter 8 cm/ Depth 4 cm

Saucer: Height 4 cm

A circular handle with a ruyi-shaped figure at its top is attached to the side of the cup. One side of the handle is embossed with a dragon while the other a phoenix, symbolizing auspiciousness. The indentation is delicate and smooth, and the spotless and bright white glaze looks translucent. The cup, with a gold-and-silver-bound ring foot, has an inscription of "Xin Guan" carved on the bottom. The saucer, with a silver-bound mouth rim and ring foot, has a "Xin Guan" mark incised on the base.

Preserved in Li'nan Museum of Cultural Relics

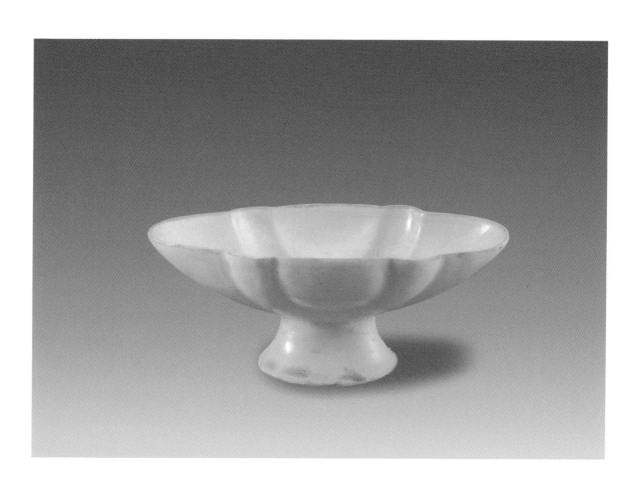

白瓷海棠杯

唐

瓷质

口长 16.1 厘米，口宽 7.8 厘米，高 6.3 厘米

White Crabapple-shaped Cup

Tang Dynasty

Porcelain

Mouth Length 16.1 cm/ Mouth Width 7.8 cm/ Depth 6.3 cm

杯口平面呈椭圆形，菱花口，似一朵盛开的海棠花。用内模坯成型，造型精巧。底刻一"官"字。在晚唐白瓷中，如此精美的作品传世甚少。1980 年临安区唐水邱氏墓出土。

临安市文物馆藏

The plane of the mouth is oval with rhombus-shaped rim resembling a white crabapple in its full blossom. The cup is delicately designed and formed by insert moulding. There is an inscription "Guan" carved on the base. Works of such delicate white porcelain from the late Tang Dynasty are rarely found today. It was unearthed at the Tang-dynasty Shuiqiu tomb in Lin'an District, Zhejiang Province, in 1980.

Preserved in Lin'an Museum of Cultural Relics

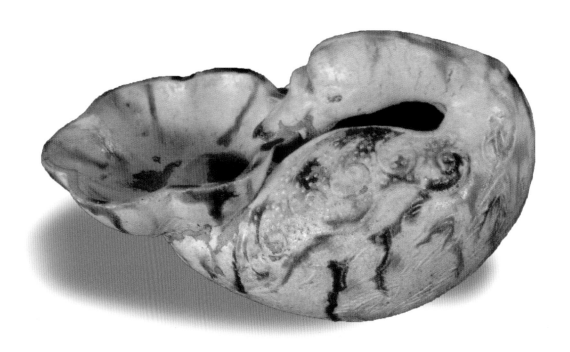

三彩鸭形杯

唐

瓷质

高 7 厘米

Tricolour Duck-shaped Cup

Tang Dynasty

Porcelain

Height 7 cm

胎呈白色。杯作卧鸭回首衔尾状，鸭长嘴，弯颈，尾作荷叶状杯口，姿态优雅柔美。杯口内外和鸭身施黄、白、绿、褐色釉，色调淡雅柔和。

河北博物院藏

The body of the cup is white. The cup is shaped into a lying duck turning back to reach the tail with its beak. The elegant and beautiful duck has a long beak and an arched neck, with a lotus-leave-shaped tail functioning as the mouth of the cup. Both the interior and exterior of the cup as well as the duck are glazed yellow, white, green and brown, the tone of which is elegant and soft.

Preserved in Hebei Museum

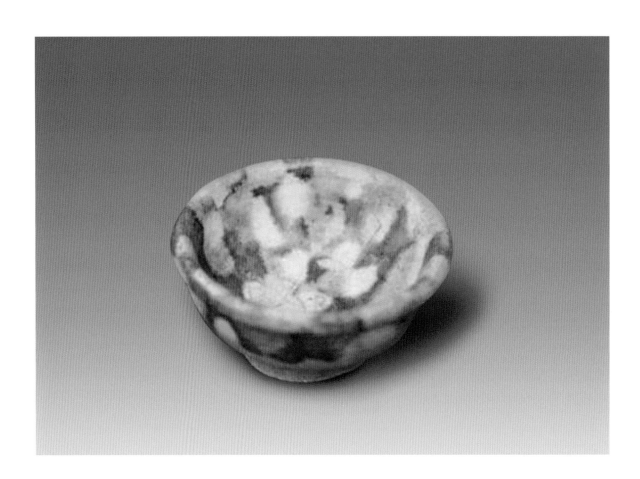

三彩小碟

唐

瓷质

外口径 5.3 厘米，底径 2.1 厘米，通高 2.3 厘米，腹深 1.65 厘米，重 31 克

Tricolour Saucer

Tang Dynasty

Porcelain

Mouth Outer Diameter 5.3 cm/ Bottom Diameter 2.1 cm/ Height 2.3 cm/ Depth 1.65 cm/ Weight 31 g

圈足，三彩，平底，口沿圆润。唐代三彩陶器的简称。明器。

广东中医药博物馆藏

The saucer has a ring foot, a flat base and a smooth mouth rim. This tricolour glazed ware is a burial object.

Preserved in Guangdong Chinese Medicine Museum

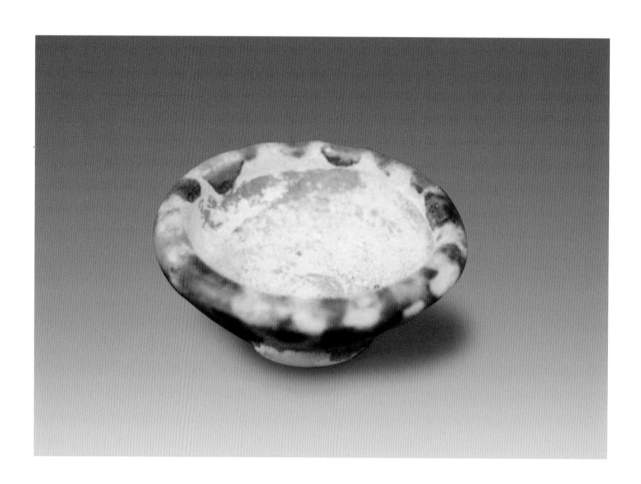

三彩小碟

唐

瓷质

外口径 5.2 厘米，底径 2.4 厘米，通高 2.3 厘米，腹深 1.7 厘米，重 35 克

Tricolour Saucer

Tang Dynasty

Porcelain

Mouth Outer Diameter 5.2 cm/ Bottom Diameter 2.4 cm/ Height 2.3 cm/ Depth 1.7 cm/ Weight 35 g

圈足，三彩，平底，口沿圆润。唐代三彩陶器的简称。明器。

广东中医药博物馆藏

The saucer has a ring foot and a flat base with a smooth mouth rim. This tricolour glazed ware is a burial object.

Preserved in Guangdong Chinese Medicine Museum

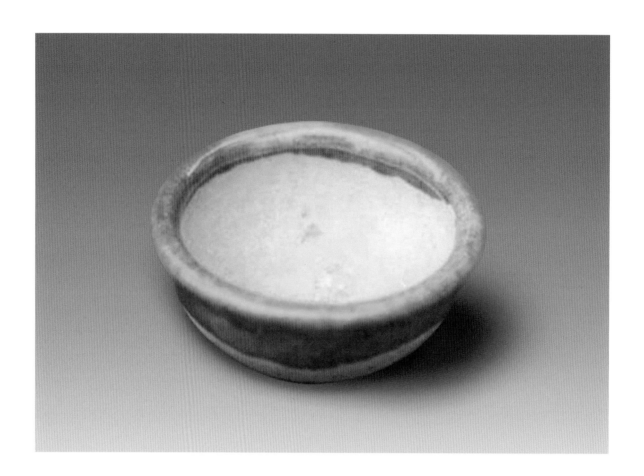

三彩小碟

唐

瓷质

外口径 5.1 厘米，底径 2.7 厘米，通高 2.3 厘米，腹深 1.9 厘米，重 35 克

Tricolour Saucer

Tang Dynasty

Porcelain

Mouth Outer Diameter 5.1 cm/ Bottom Diameter 2.7 cm/ Height 2.3 cm/ Depth 1.9 cm/ Weight 35 g

平底，口沿圆润。三彩，唐代三彩陶器的简称。
明器。

广东中医药博物馆藏

The saucer has a flat base and a smooth mouth rim. This tricolour glazed ware is a burial object.

Preserved in Guangdong Chinese Medicine Museum

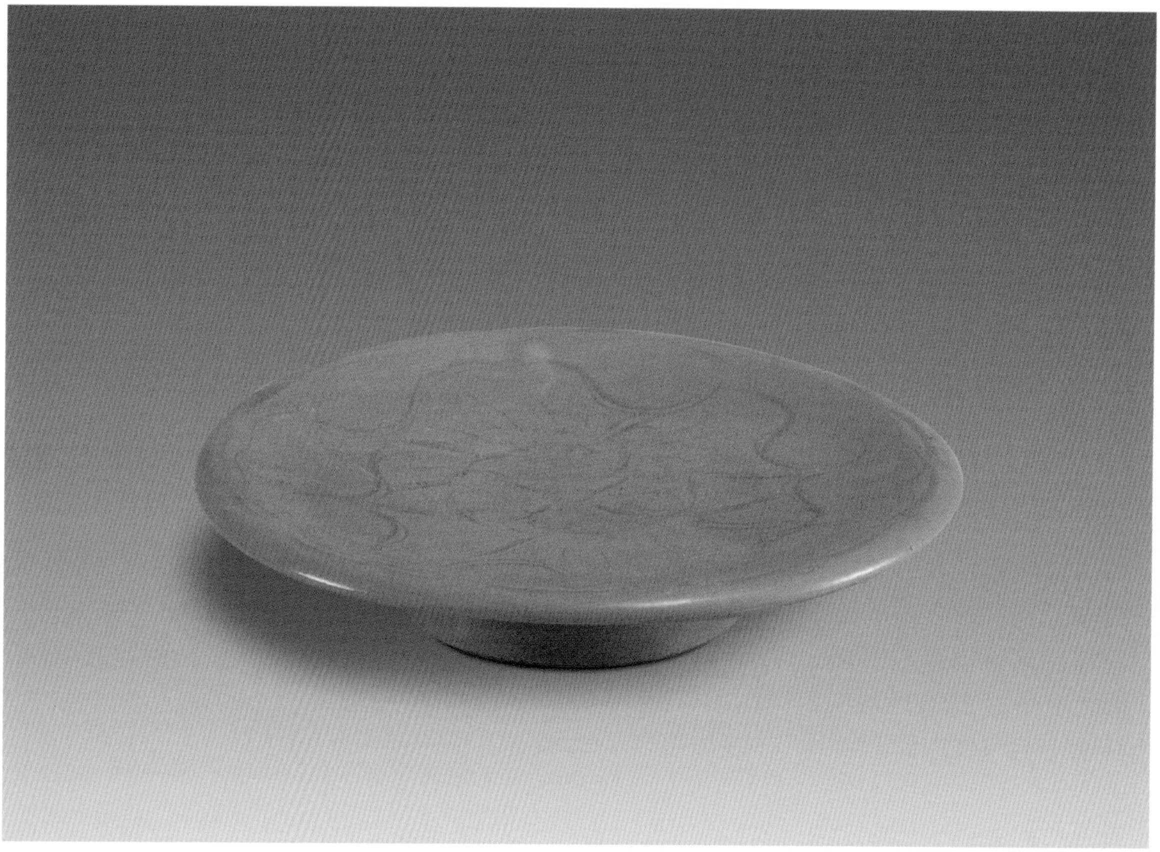

碟

唐

瓷质

口径 10.2 厘米，高 2.2 厘米

Plate

Tang Dynasty

Porcelain

Mouth Diameter 10.2 cm/ Height 2.2 cm

整器较矮，碟面较平，刻画荷叶纹，圈足略高，外腹压出四道短痕，满青釉泛黄，足底刮釉，有 7 个泥点痕。1994 年慈溪市上林湖荷花蕊窑址出土。

浙江省文物考古研究所藏

With a relatively high ring foot, the plate is comparatively short with lotus leaves carved on the flat surface and four short curves pressed on the outside of the stomach. The plate is covered with yellowish-green glaze, except the foot rim. There are seven mud spots on the base. It was unearthed from Lianhuarui kiln site by Shanglin Lake of Cixi City, Zhejiang Province, in the year 1994.

Preserved in Institute of Cultural Relics and Archaeology of Zhejiang Province

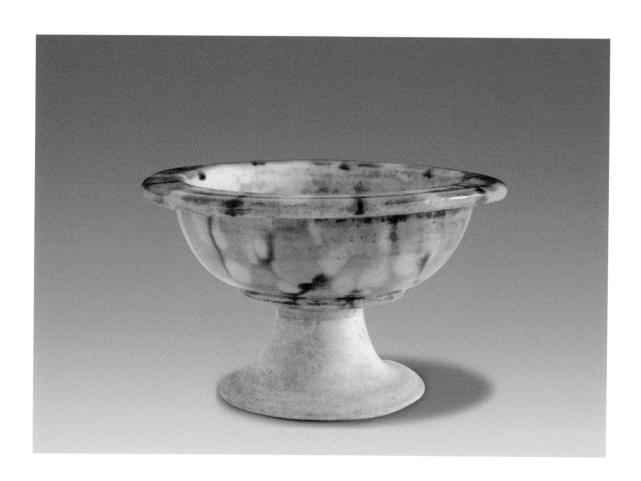

三彩豆

唐

瓷质

口径 10.4 厘米，底径 6.1 厘米，高 6.1 厘米

Tricolour Food Container

Tang Dynasty

Porcelain

Mouth Diameter 10.4 cm/ Bottom Diameter 6.1 cm/ Height 6.1 cm

敞口，折沿，弧形腹，高足外撇。折沿至腹外部施褐、黄、白、绿釉，腹内及足不施釉，釉色莹润，清淡得宜。

邓君堂藏

The container has a flared mouth, a flanged mouth rim, a bow-shaped belly and a high ring foot which gradually widens. The area from the mouth rim to the exterior body is glazed brown, yellow, white and green, while the interior body and foot are left unglazed. The glaze is bright and smooth with all the colours perfectly matched.

Collected by Deng Juntang

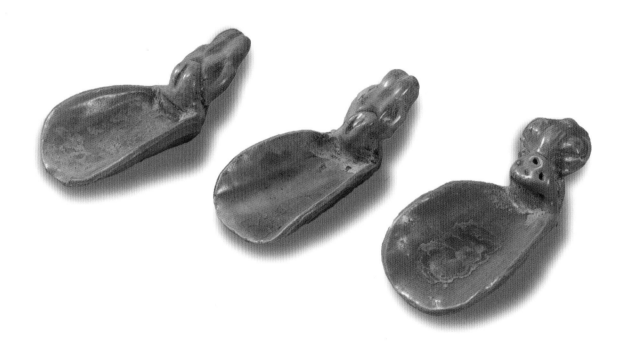

匙

唐

瓷质

长 4.8 厘米

勺体相近，把做成各种形状。满青釉，底刮釉。

浙江省文物考古研究所藏

Spoon

Tang Dynasty

Porcelain

Length 4.8 cm

The bodies of the spoons in this set are similar in shape, but the handles varies widely in design. The bodies are glazed green with the base unglazed.

Preserved in Institute of Cultural Relics and Archaeology of Zhejiang Province

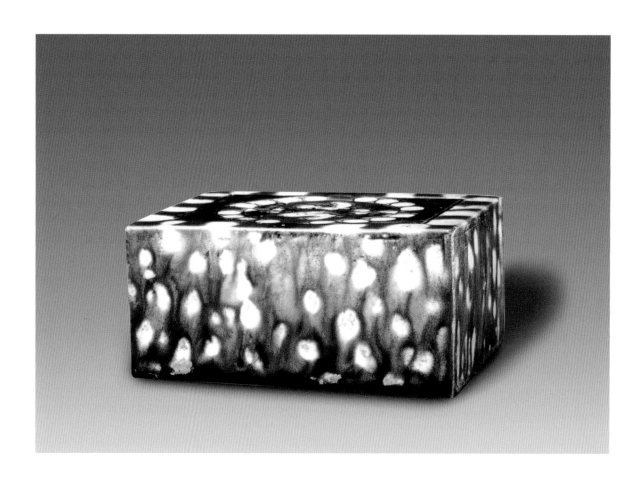

三彩双鸭方枕

唐

瓷质

长 11.2 厘米，宽 9.7 厘米，高 5.2 厘米

Tricolour Rectangular Pillow with Double Duck Design

Tang Dynasty

Porcelain

Length 11.2 cm/ Width 9.7 cm/ Height 5.2 cm

长方形，是唐代常见枕式。枕面及边壁施黄、绿、白三彩釉，底部无釉露胎。枕面长方形开光，内刻画双鸭对首展翅图，周围辅忍冬纹，开光外有一周圆珠纹边饰。

故宫博物院藏

The rectangular pillow is commonly seen in the Tang dynasty. Its face and walls are glazed yellow, green and white with the bottom unglazed. On the top of the pillow is incised a rectangular recessed panel, ornamented with bead pattern edge, within which is carved a design of two head-on ducks waving their wings, surrounded with lonicera waves.

Preserved in the Palace Museum

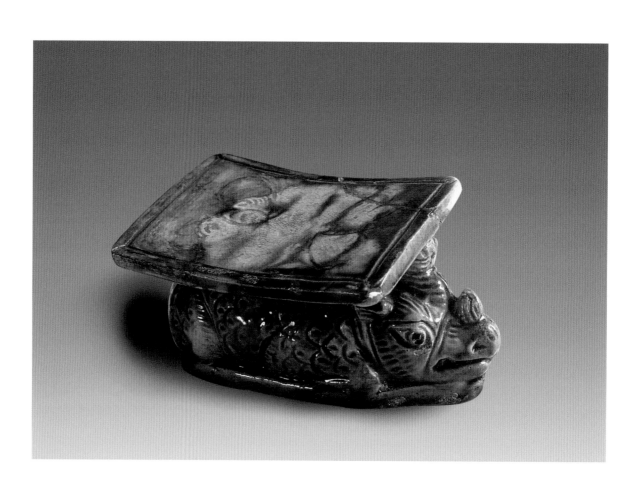

三彩犀牛枕

唐

瓷质

长 11.2 厘米，宽 8.4 厘米，高 7.5 厘米

Tricolour Rhino-shaped Pillow

Tang Dynasty

Porcelain

Length 11.2 cm/ Width 8.4 cm/ Height 7.5 cm

枕面作长方形，微弧凹，中间刻一对同向展翅飞翔的蝴蝶，边缘一周阴刻线。枕座为匍匐的犀牛伏于托子上。底露砖红胎，胎质坚硬。有三个支钉垫烧痕迹。犀牛是生活在热带地区的动物，形体硕大、健壮、凶悍、形象怪异，犀角是珍贵的药材。此枕的所有者期望用该枕能驱病避邪，降服妖魔，身体安康。1985 年扬州教育学院工地出土。

扬州博物馆藏

The rectangular pillow face is slightly concave, with a pair of butterflies flying in the same direction carved in the centre, enclosed by a circle of incised lines on the edge. The lower part of the pillow is in the shape of a rhino crawling on the base. The hard red brick body is exposed on the bottom with three spur marks for firing on it. A rhino is a strong, large and fierce animal living in tropical areas. Though it looks monstrous, its horn can be used as precious medicinal herbs. The owner of this pillow wanted to use it to ward off diseases and evil spirits, thus ensuring good health. It was unearthed at the construction site of Yangzhou Education College, Jiangsu Province, in 1985.

Preserved in Yangzhou Museum

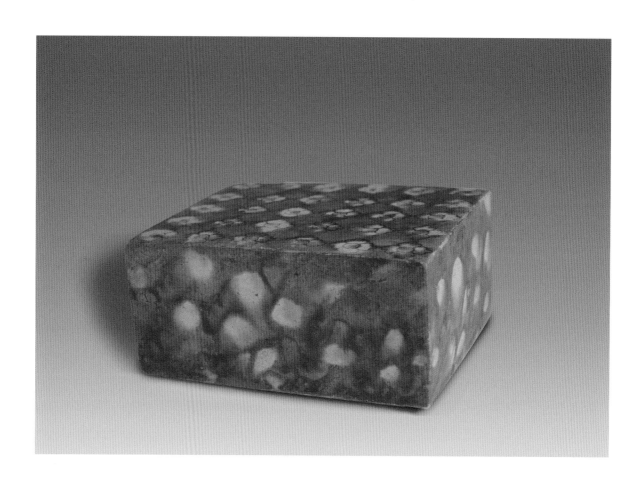

三彩枕

唐

瓷质

长 10.3 厘米，宽 8.6 厘米，高 4.5 厘米

Tricolour Pillow

Tang Dynasty

Porcelain

Length 10.3 cm/ Width 8.6 cm/ Height 4.5 cm

枕为日字方形，六面满施彩釉，四侧面为黄、绿、白相间斑釉，两面绘梅花朵纹，彩色莹润。绿、黄、白三色相映，争妍斗胜，瑰丽异常。釉里现极细小的纹片，是盛唐时期的代表作。

颂德藏

The pillow is of cuboid form with six sides glazed colourfully. On the four vertical sides is mottled enamel in yellow, green and white colours alternatively; while on the top and the bottom are painted bright and smooth plum blossom patterns in perfectly matched green, yellow and white colours. As very tiny crackles are found in the glaze, it is a representative piece of the High Tang Period.

Collected by Song De

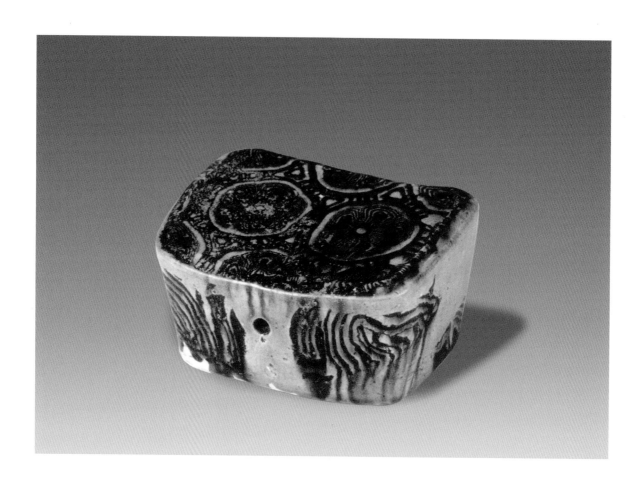

绿釉搅胎枕

唐

瓷质

长 14.3 厘米，宽 10.9 厘米，高 7.7 厘米

Green-glazed Pillow with Twisted Clay

Tang Dynasty

Porcelain

Length 14.3 cm/ Width 10.9 cm/ Height 7.7 cm

枕面两端稍高，中间微凹，略呈马鞍状。枕体中空，前壁有一圆形小孔。枕面及枕壁均用搅胎装饰，枕面为变体莲花纹，枕壁为木理纹。纹饰自然流畅，并施绿釉，枕底露胎。此枕系巩县窑产品。1975年扬州双桥乡卜桥村出土。

扬州博物馆藏

The pillow face is in the shape of a saddle with both ends slightly higher and the middle concave. It is hollow inside with a round hole in the front wall. Both the pillow face and the walls, incised naturally and smoothly with variant lotus patterns and wood veins respectively, are decorated with twisted clay. The body is glazed green with the bottom unglazed. This pillow is a porcelain product from Gongxian County Kiln, unearthed in Puqiao Village in Shuangqiao Township of Yangzhou, Jiangsu Province, in the year 1975. Preserved in Yangzhou Museum

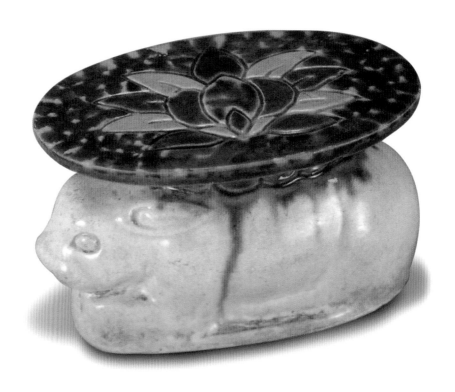

三彩卧兔枕

唐

瓷质

长 12.1 厘米，宽 8 厘米，高 7.3 厘米

Tricolour Lying-rabbit-shaped Pillow

Tang Dynasty

Porcelain

Length 12.1 cm/ Width 8cm/ Height 7.3 cm

胎质洁白细腻，敷白色化妆土，枕作卧兔状，兔睁目伸耳，伏卧于椭圆形座板上，背承椭圆形枕面。枕面刻一莲花，上施蓝、绿、褐三色釉。

河北博物院藏

The pillow, whose white and fine body is coated with white engobe, is in the shape of a rabbit lying on an oval base with round eyes and stretched ears. On the back of the rabbit is a oval-shaped pillow face, on which is carved a lotus with blue, green and brown glaze.

Preserved in Hebei Museum

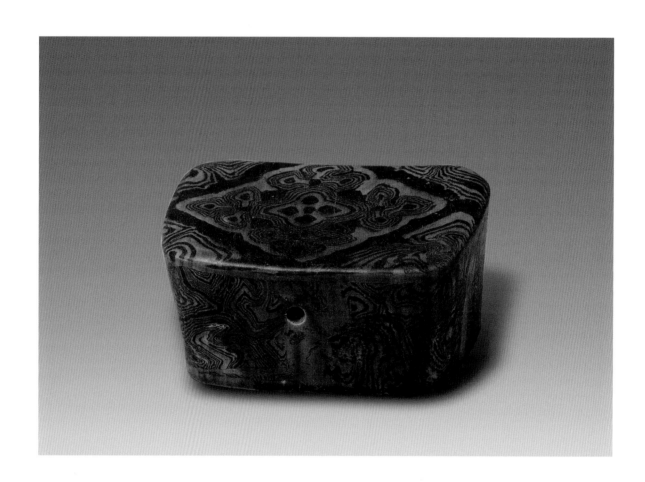

绿釉绞胎枕

唐

瓷质

长 16 厘米，宽 10.8 厘米，高 8 厘米

Green-glazed Pillow with Twisted Clay

Tang Dynasty

Porcelain

Length 16 cm/ Width 10.8 cm/ Height 8 cm

白胎，施豆绿色釉。枕略作长方体，枕面微凹，一侧有小圆孔。底为白胎，枕面及四侧面由白、赭两色泥料绞制而成，用赭色泥料组成菱形纹及木纹，菱形内饰梅朵纹。绞胎陶瓷盛行于唐末，多为河南瓷窑烧制，纹理清晰，自然雅致。1987 年兖州市李海村出土。

兖州博物馆藏

The white pillow body is glazed pea green. The cuboid pillow face is slightly concave with a small hole on one side. The white body is exposed on the bottom, and the face and the four sides are made of twisted clay in the combination of white and ocher colours. Wood vein patterns of the ocher clay and a plum buds motif enclosed in rhombus forms can be found. Porcelain wares with twisted clay, natural and elegant with clear vein patterns, were prevalent in the late Tang dynasty and were mostly fired in kilns in Henan Province. This pillow was unearthed in Lihai Village of Yanzhou, Jiangsu Province, in the year 1987.

Preserved in Yanzhou Museum

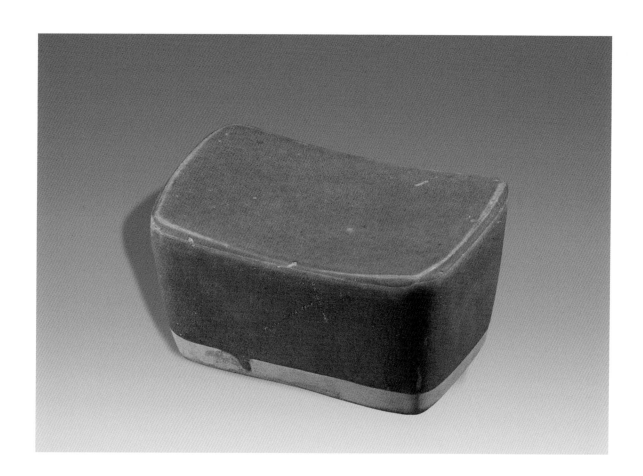

长沙窑绿釉枕

唐

瓷质

长 13.9 厘米，宽 9.3 厘米，高 6.2~6.9 厘米

Green-glazed Pillow from Changsha Kiln

Tang Dynasty

Porcelain

Length 13.9 cm/ Width 9.3 cm/ Height 6.2–6.9 cm

枕形近长方体，倭角，枕面下凹。施绿色釉，
釉面开细小纹片，釉薄处可见胎色。底露胎，
胎质粉白略显灰黄色，后壁转角处有一出气孔。

常州博物馆藏

The pillow, glazed green with tiny crackles,
is of cuboid form with rounded corners and
concave face. The white and slightly greyish
yellow body can be seen where the glaze is thin
and the body is exposed on the bottom. There is
a vent hole in the corner of the back wall.

Preserved in Changzhou Museum

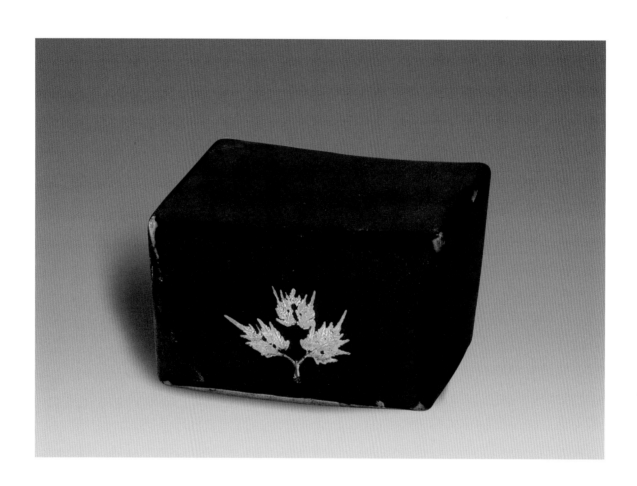

茶末釉贴花枕

唐

瓷质

长 12.8 厘米，宽 10.4 厘米，高 8.6 厘米

Tea-flake-glazed Pillow with Applique Decoration

Tang Dynasty

Porcelain

Length 12.8 cm/ Width 10.4 cm/ Height 8.6 cm

枕作长方形，枕面两端稍高，面微弧凹。枕件中空，侧壁有一圆形小孔。前、后壁各贴一片枫叶，再施灰褐色茶叶末釉，烧结后形成露胎的枫叶图案。枕底露胎，胎灰白细腻，为寿州窑产品。1980 年工凤砖瓦厂出土。

扬州博物馆藏

The pillow face is rectangular with both ends slightly higher and the middle a little concave. It is hollow inside with a small hole in the wall. Two applique maple leaves were attached to the front and back walls respectively and then coated with taupe tea-flake glaze. The maple leaf pattern was thus formed after firing. The fine and smooth greyish white body is exposed on the bottom. It is a product from Shouzhou kiln and was unearthed at Gongfeng Brick and Tile Plant in the year 1980.

Preserved in Yangzhou Museum

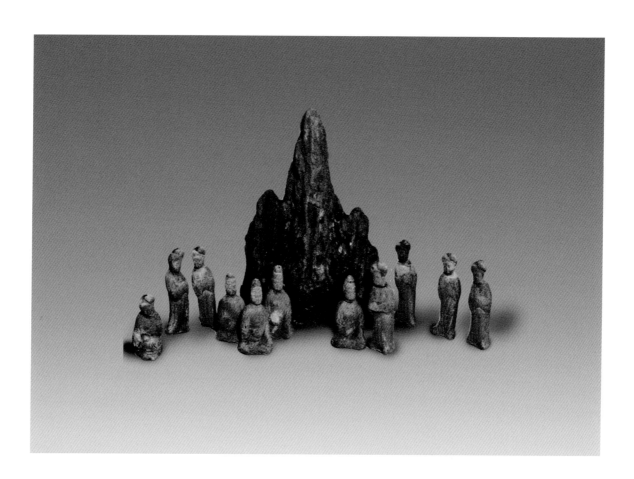

加彩游山人物俑

唐

瓷质

彩山：高 23.4 厘米

Painted Figurines of Mountain-hikers

Tang Dynasty

Porcelain

Mountain: Height 23.4 cm

游山是古代人们进行户外娱乐活动的主要形式
之一。这里展示的一组包括男女 12 人的游山
人物俑群，真实地再现了当时人们进行户外游
山活动的情景。

陕西历史博物馆藏

Mountain hiking is one of the main outdoor
recreation activities for the ancient people.
This set of exhibition, including 12 female and
male figurines, vividly portrays the scene of
mountain hiking back then.

Preserved Shaanxi Museum of Medical History

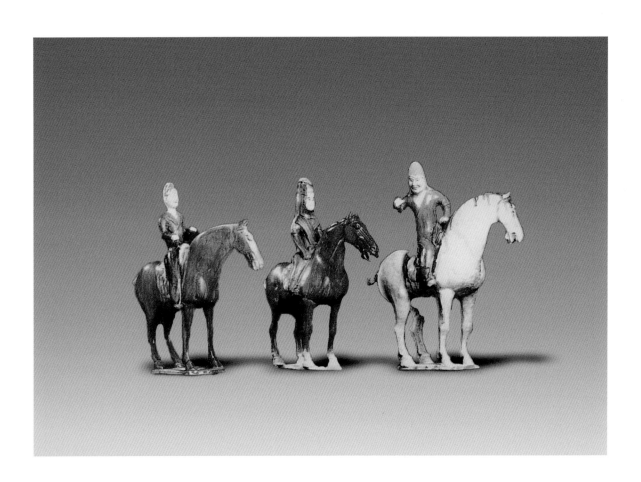

三彩骑马出游俑

唐

瓷质

高 36.5~41 厘米

Tricolour Figurine of Equestrians on Sightseeing

Tang Dynasty

Porcelain

Height 36.5–41 cm

在唐代，策骑出游是时人喜爱的一项户外娱乐活动。这三件三彩骑马出游俑之中，其一为仕女，一为随员，一为领队。马皆立足昂首。领队骑者正在拉停马，回首向仕女讲述行程。此三彩俑的造型，颇具生活情趣。

徐氏艺术馆藏

In the Tang Dynasty, riding was a popular outdoor recreational activity. This set includes three tricolour figurines: a lady, an entourage and a leader, and three horses standing firmly on the pedestal with their heads up. The leader seems like stopping his horse, turning around to the lady and telling her about the planned schedule. The design of these tricolour figurines is very vivid.

Preserved in Tsui Museum of Art

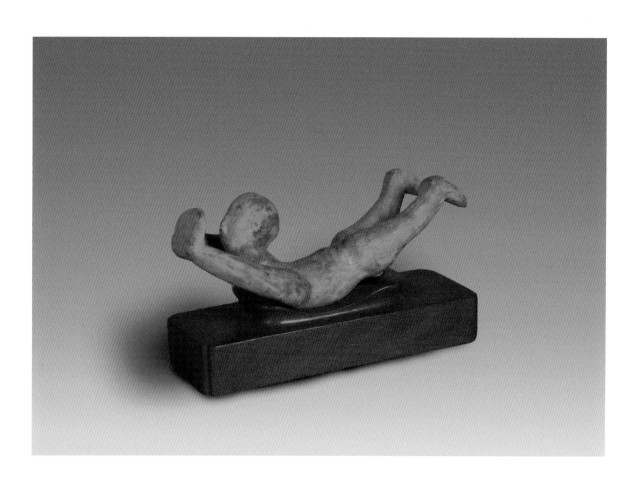

游泳陶俑

唐

陶质

通高 9.3 厘米，宽 4 厘米

Pottery Figurine of a Swimmer

Tang Dynasty

Pottery

Height 9.3 cm/ Width 4 cm

浅棕黄色，人物为男性，作游泳状。明器。

1955 年入藏。保存基本完好。

中华医学会 / 上海中医药大学医史博物馆藏

This pottery figurine is a male swimmer in light brown colour. This burial object, collected in 1955, is well preserved.

Preserved in Chinese Medical Association/Museum of Chinese Medicine, Shanghai University of Traditional Chinese Medicine

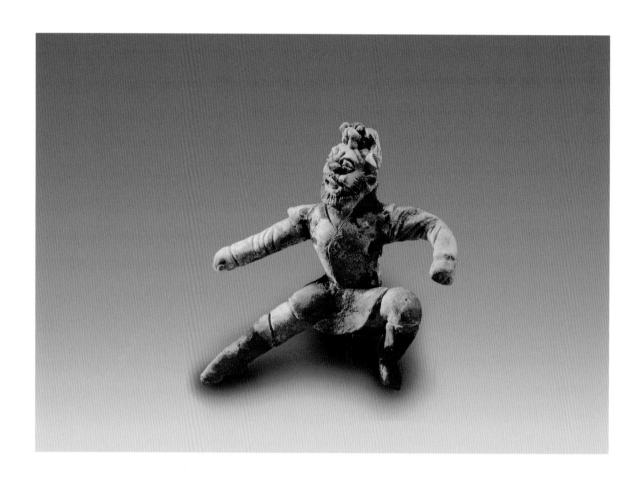

彩绘习武泥俑

唐

泥质

高 10.2 厘米

Painted Figurine of a Warrior Practicing Martial Arts

Tang Dynasty

Clay

Height 10.2 cm

俑为豹目，狮鼻，连鬓短须，应是一胡人武士形象。其双手握拳，双臂微弓；左腿下蹲，呈弓状，右腿向右斜伸，表现的正是武士进行拳术演练的一个瞬间动作。1960 年新疆维吾尔自治区吐鲁番市阿斯塔那 336 号唐墓出土。

新疆维吾尔自治区博物馆藏

This pottery figurine resembles a Mongols from the countries west of China, with leopard-like eyes, a pug nose, sideburns and short beards. He clenches his fists, slightly bends his arms, squats with his left leg bent like a bow, and stretches his right leg towards the right. It portrays a moment when the warrior is practicing the Chinese boxing. It was unearthed at No. 336 Tang Dynasty Tomb at Astana in Turpan City, Xinjiang Uygur Autonomous Region, in the year 1960.
Preserved in Xinjiang Uygur Autonomous Region Museum

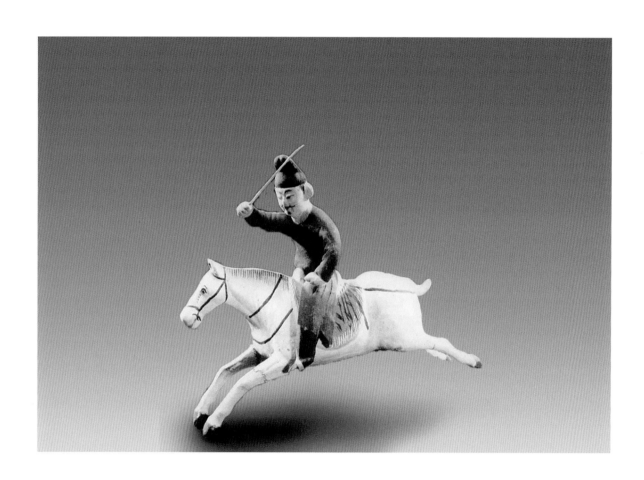

彩绘打马球泥俑

唐

泥质

通高 37 厘米

Painted Clay Figurine of an Equestrian Polo Player

Tang Dynasty

Clay

Height 37 cm

泥俑黄泥成型，所着色彩和墨线都基本完好。击球者身穿紫色圆领长袍，头戴尖顶帽，足蹬黑靴，正骑在四蹄腾起的奔马上挥杖击球，成功地再现了唐代边疆地区马球活动盛况。1972年新疆维吾尔自治区吐鲁番市阿斯塔那230号唐墓出土。

新疆维吾尔自治区博物馆藏

The colours and ink sketch of the figurine, made of yellow clay, are largely intact. The man, in a purple round-collar robe, with a peaked cap on his head and a pair of black boots on the feet, is waving the rod to hit the ball on a galloping horse. The clay figurine vividly portrays the spectacular scene of a polo match in border areas in the Tang dynasty. It was unearthed from No. 230 Tang Dynasty Tomb at Astana in Turpan City, Xinjiang Uygur Autonomous Region, in 1972.

Preserved in Xinjiang Uygur Autonomous Region Museum

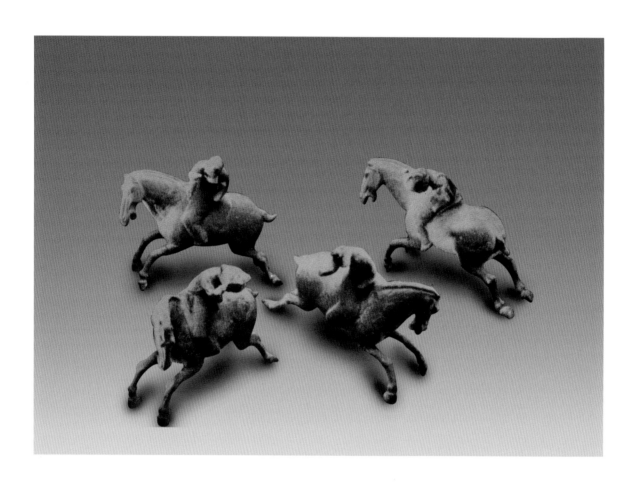

彩绘骑马击球陶俑群

唐

陶质

高约 25.4 厘米

Painted Pottery Figurines of Polo Equestrian Hitting the Ball

Tang Dynasty

Pottery

Height 25.4 cm

这是 1948 年由夏蕙·姬丝汀女士赞助购藏的四件击球俑。击球者的坐骑均呈四蹄跃起状，女骑手们正全神贯注地俯身击球。

美国肯萨斯市纳尔逊·雅坚斯美术博物馆藏

This set of four figurines was collected in 1984 with the sponsorship of Mrs. Sherry Christine. The horses of the ball-hitters are all running so fast that their hooves leave the ground. The female riders are absorbedly bending over to hit the ball.

Preserved in Nelson-Artkins Museum of Art, Kansas City, U.S.A.

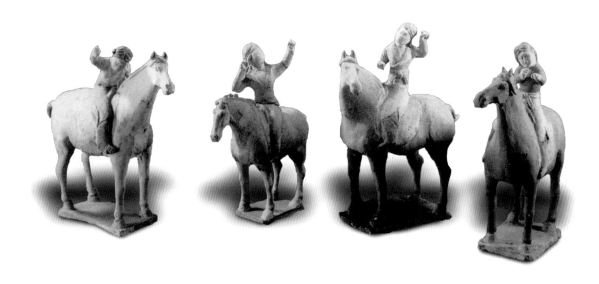

彩绘打马球陶俑群

唐

陶质

通高 30 ~ 33.5 厘米

Painted Pottery Figurines of Polo Equestrians

Tang Dynasty

Pottery

Height 30–33.5 cm

这组打马球俑共 4 件，均为陶质彩绘。马身彩绘鲜艳夺目，呈昂首直立状，骑在马上的击球者，均头梳双髻，身穿红、绿色翻领外衣和骑士裤，足踏黑靴，神情专注地做各种击球的姿势。1959 年陕西省长安区南里王村唐韦炯墓出土。

陕西历史博物馆藏

This group of pottery polo equestrian consists of four painted pieces. The horses, coated with beautifully-coloured painting, raise their heads high and stand upright. The players on the horses, with two buns on their heads, all wear red and green lapel jackets, knight's pants and black boots, attentively making all kinds of poses to hit the polo. It was excavated in the tomb of Tang Weijiong in Nan Liwang Village of Chang'an District in Xi'an, Shaanxi Province in 1959.

Preserved in shaanxi History Museum

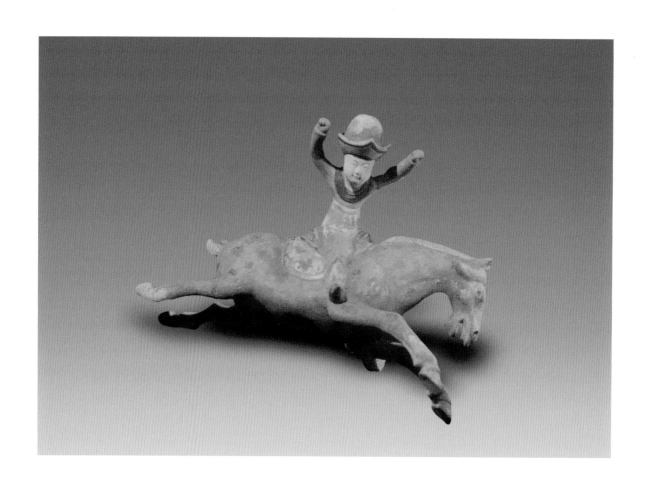

彩绘描金击球俑

唐

陶质

长 37.8 厘米，高 23.3 厘米

Painted Figurine of a Polo Equestrienne in Gold Tracery

Tang Dynasty

Pottery

Length 37.8 cm/ Height 23.3 cm

此为击球俑中的传世精品。击球者为一女子，

身骑四蹄跃起的奔马，正全神贯注地俯身击球，

成功地再现了马球运动的瞬间动态。

上海博物馆藏

The female rider on the galloping horse is
absorbedly bending over to hit the ball. A
masterpiece of its kind, the figurine reproduces
the momentary motion of the polo sport.

Preserved in Shanghai Museum

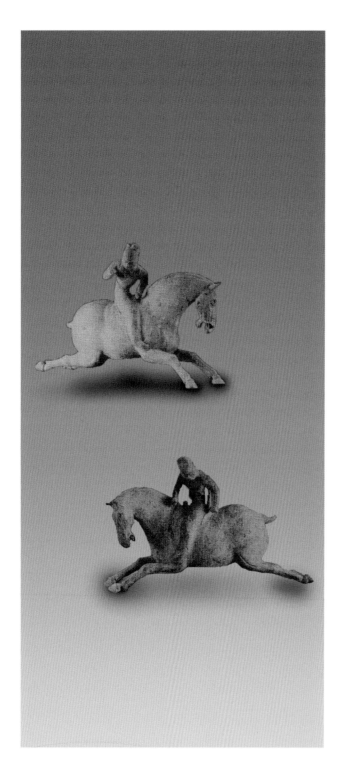

彩绘打马球陶俑

唐

陶质

高 40~41 厘米

Painted Pottery Figurines of Polo Equestrians

Tang Dynasty

Pottery

Height 40–41 cm

两头发结成双髻的骑士，正骑在呈奔跑状的马上弯身击球。奔马张口，头向左倾。两俑对击球人物和健骑刻画的甚为精细，表现了勇士们策马争球的激烈场面。

徐氏艺术馆藏

Two riders with two-bun hairstyle are riding galloping horses and bending over to hit the ball. The heads of the running horses are inclined to the left with their mouths open. The exquisite sculptures of the polo players and the muscular horses vividly portray the intense scene of the warriors vying with one another for the ball.

Preserved in Tsui Museum of Art

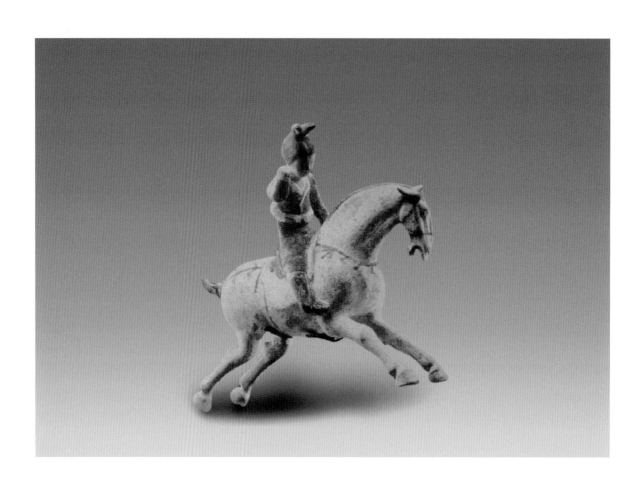

彩绘打马球俑

唐

陶质

高 35 厘米

Painted Figurine of a Polo Equestrienne

Tang Dynasty

Pottery

Height 35 cm

该马球俑，饰以彩绘，造型为女骑手呈右臂挥舞球杖做击球状，成功地再现了马球竞赛的瞬间动态。此为击球俑。

法国吉美国立亚洲艺术博物馆藏

The painted polo equestrienne is swinging the shooting cane with her right arm to hit the ball, portraying vividly an instantaneous motion during a polo match. This is a figurine of a polo hitter.

Preserved in Musée National des Arts Asiatiques-Guimet, France

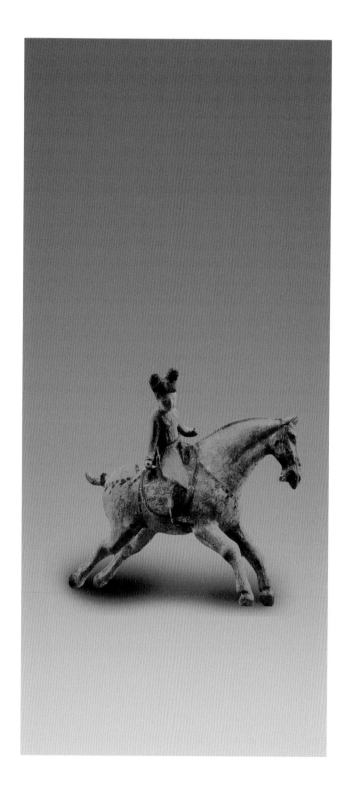

彩绘打马球俑

唐

陶质

高 31 厘米

Painted Figurine of a Polo Equestrienne

Tang Dynasty

Pottery

Height 31 cm

该马球俑，饰以彩绘，造型为头梳双髻女骑手，左手持缰绳，右手持杖，双眼凝视着球，成功地再现了马球竞赛的精彩瞬间。此为击球俑。

法国吉美国立亚洲艺术博物馆藏

This painted polo figurine is a female player with double topknots, whose left hand is holding the rein, while in the right hand is the shooting cane. Her eyes are gazing at the ball. The figurine vividly portrays the exciting moment during a polo match. This is a figurine of a polo hitter. This is a pottery figurine of polo-hitter.

Preserved in Musée National des Arts Asiatiques-Guimet, France

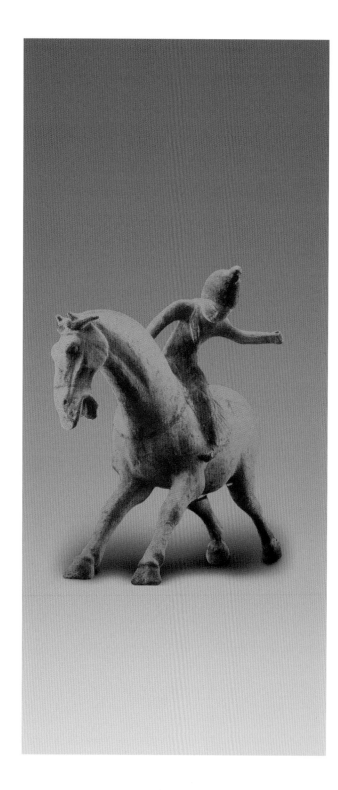

彩绘打马球俑

唐

陶质

高 31 厘米

Painted Figurine of a Polo Equestrienne

Tang Dynasty

Pottery

Height 31cm

该马球俑，饰以彩绘，造型为女骑手，呈左臂
挥舞球杖，做俯身击球状，成功地再现了马球
竞赛的瞬间动态。此为击球俑。

法国吉美国立亚洲艺术博物馆藏

The painted polo equestrienne is swinging the
shooting cane with her left arm, and is bending
down to hit the ball, portraying vividly an
instantaneous motion of a polo match. This is a
figurine of a polo hitter.

Preserved in Musée National des Arts Asiatiques-
Guimet, France

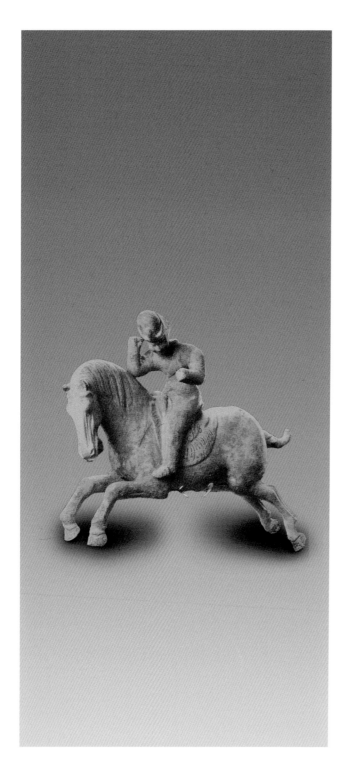

彩绘打马球俑

唐

陶质

高 36 厘米

Painted Figurine of a Polo Equestrienne

Tang Dynasty

Pottery

Height 36 cm

该马球俑，饰以彩绘，造型为骑手俯身击球状，成功展现了马球竞赛的精彩瞬间。此为击球俑。

法国吉美国立亚洲艺术博物馆藏

The painted polo equestrienne is bending down to hit the ball, portraying vividly an instantaneous motion during a polo match. This is a figurine of a polo hitter.

Preserved in Musée National des Arts Asiatiques-Guimet, France

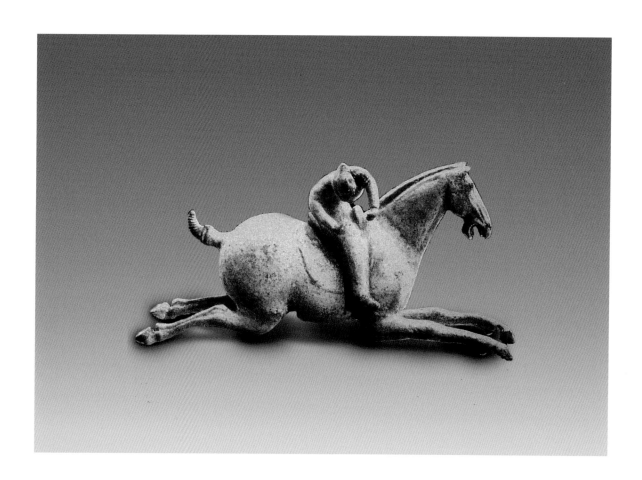

彩绘打马球俑

唐
陶质
高 26 厘米

Painted Figurine of a Polo Equestrienne

Tang Dynasty
Pottery
Height 26 cm

该马球俑，饰以彩绘，造型为骑手，呈疾驰挥右臂击球状，成功地再现了马球竞赛的精彩瞬间。此为击球俑。

法国吉美国立亚洲艺术博物馆藏

This painted polo figurine is a rider, who is swinging his right arm, hitting the ball on the galloping horse. The polo hitter figurine successfully portrays the exciting moment during a polo match. This is a pottery figurine of a polo-hitter.

Preserved in Musée National des Arts Asiatiques-Guimet, France

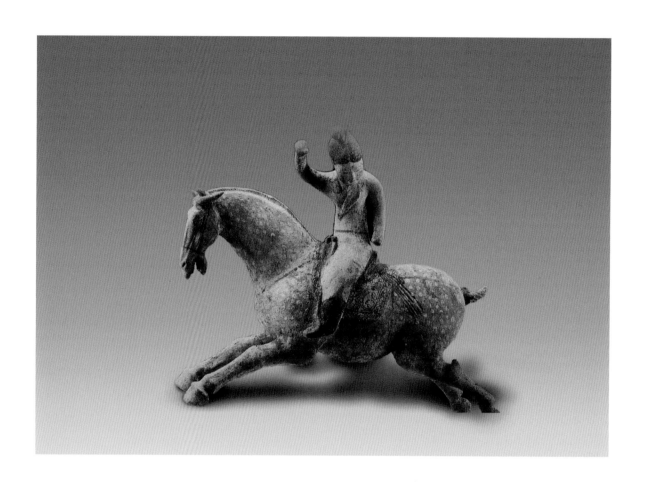

彩绘打马球俑

唐

陶质

高 32 厘米

Painted Figurine of a Polo Equestrienne

Tang Dynasty

Pottery

Height 32 cm

该马球俑，饰以彩绘，造型为女骑手，右臂挥舞做击球状，再现了马球竞赛的精彩瞬间。此为击球俑。

法国吉美国立亚洲艺术博物馆藏

The painted polo figurine is a female player, whose right arm is swung out to hit the ball. The figurine vividly portrays the exciting moment during a polo match. This is a figurine of a polo hitter. This is a pottery figurine of a polo-hitter. Preserved in Musée National des Arts Asiatiques-Guimet, France

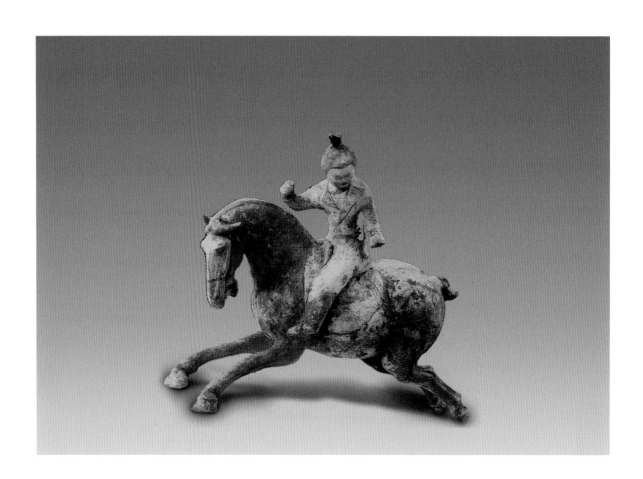

彩绘打马球俑

唐

陶质

高 30 厘米

Painted Figurine of a Polo Equestrienne

Tang Dynasty

Pottery

Height 30 cm

一套共 6 件，均饰以彩绘，造型皆为伏身在奔马上做右臂挥舞球杖的击球动作。此为其中的击球俑之一。

法国罗杰·阿森伯格藏

This set of polo figurines includes six painted pieces all moulded into riders on galloping horses in the pose of waving ball rods with their right arms to hit the ball. This object is one of the pottery figurines of a polo-hitter.

Collected by Roger Ahrensburg, France

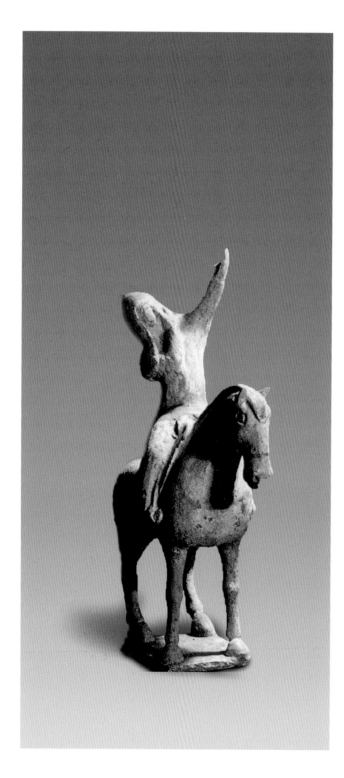

骑射陶俑

唐

陶质

高约 35 厘米

Pottery Figurine of an Equestrian Archer

Tang Dynasty

Pottery

Height 35 cm

这件流传至国外的陶俑，成功地塑造了一位唐代骑射武士的形象。这位武士身着铠甲，体态健壮，正在马上执弓瞄向空中的目标。

美国纽约莉莲·斯卡露丝藏

This pottery figurine which was found overseas portrays successfully the image of a equestrian archer in the Tang dynasty. Encased in armour, this muscular warrior on horseback is aiming the bow toward the target in the air.

Collected by Lilien Scaruth, U.S.A.

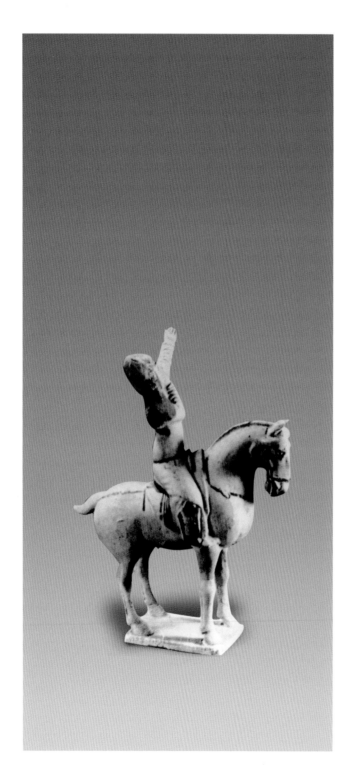

三彩陶骑射俑

唐

陶质

通高 27 厘米

Tricolour Pottery Figurine of an Equestrian Archer

Tang Dynasty

Pottery

Height 27 cm

胎呈白色。马上的骑士，头戴红色风帽，身
穿窄袖绿色长袍，足踏长筒黑靴，左臂向上
斜伸，呈拉弓状，表现了弓箭将要射出的一
刹那。1972年陕西省礼泉县唐郑仁泰墓出土。

陕西历史博物馆藏

The body of this figurine is white. The rider
on the horse wears a narrow-sleeved green
jacket, with a red cowl on his head and a pair
of long black boots on his feet. His left arm
stretches upwards as if drawing a bow, which
shows the moment when the bow is about
to speed forth. It was excavated from Zheng
Rentai tomb of the Tang Dynasty in Liquan
County, Shaanxi Province, in 1972.
Preserved in shaanxi History Museum

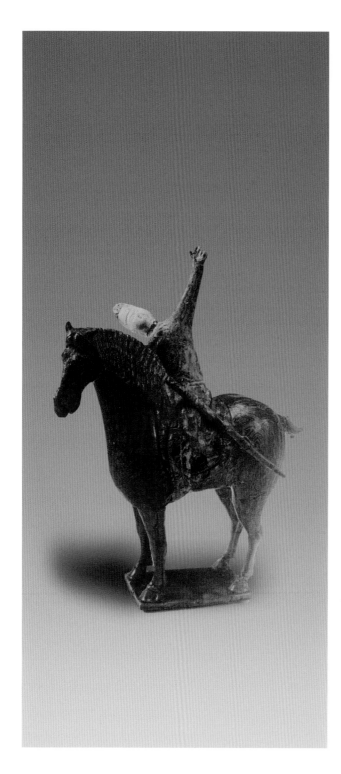

绞胎三彩骑射俑

唐

陶质

高 36.2 厘米

Tricolour Pottery Figurine of an Equestrian Archer with Twisted Clay

Tang Dynasty

Pottery

Height 36.2 cm

这件陶俑塑造了一位骑马仰射的唐代武士形象。其体态健壮，神情坚毅，正聚精会神，张弓搭箭向空中的目标瞄准。1971 年陕西省乾县唐李重润墓出土。

陕西历史博物馆藏

This pottery figurine succeeds in portraying the image of a Tang-dynasty archery warrior on horseback, who is drawing the bow upward. With a robust physique and adamant facial expression, the warrior is attentively aiming the bow at the target in the air. It was excavated from Li Chongrun tomb of the Tang Dynasty in Qian County, Shaanxi Province, in 1971. Preserved in shaanxi History Museum

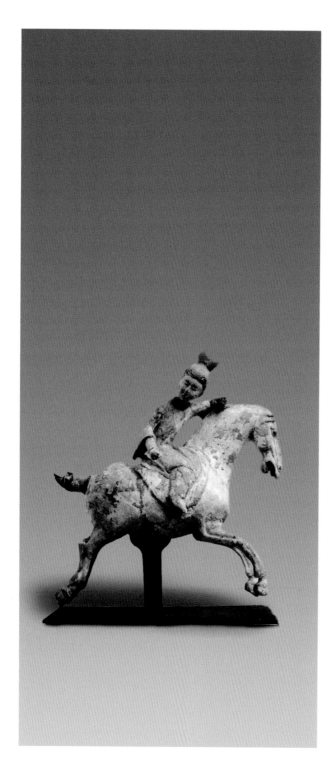

骑马俑

唐

陶质

高 30 厘米

Figurine of an Equestrienne

Tang Dynasty

Pottery

Height 30 cm

骑马俑为加彩陶质，造型表现了一女骑手骑在

马上正在作竞跑状的情景。

日本天理参考馆藏

This figurine is a pottery with paints added,
which captures the scene of a horsewoman
riding a running horse in a race.
Preserved in Tenri University Sankokan Museum

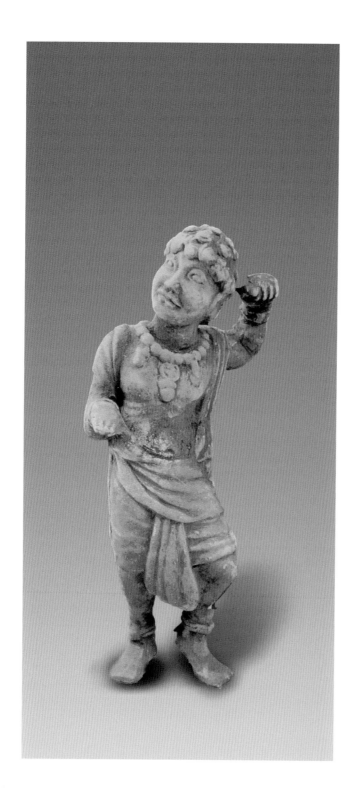

彩绘黑人舞俑

唐

陶质

宽 7.5 厘米，高 25 厘米

Painted Figurine of a Dark-skinned Dancer

Tang Dynasty

Pottery

Width 7.5 cm/ Height 25 cm

俑为昆仑形象。卷发，黑肤，赤足，高鼻，双目圆睁，面带微笑。颈饰璎珞，手腕、脚踝戴舞环。橘红丝帛绕双肩缠至下腹及膝盖上部。左臂举至头际，右手放至腰部，右腿后蹬扭胯，作舞状。

陕西省咸阳市长武县博物馆藏

The figurine shows the image of a curly-haired and high-nosed Kunlun man in dark skin who, bare-footed, smiles with eyes wide open. He wears a pearl and jade necklace with dance rings around his wrist as well as the ankle. The orange silk covers his shoulders and goes all the way down to his lower abdomen and upper knees. This figurine is dancing with his left arm upward to the head, his right hand around the waist, his right leg pushing backward and the hip twisting.

Preserved in Changwu Museum in Xianyang, Shaanxi Province

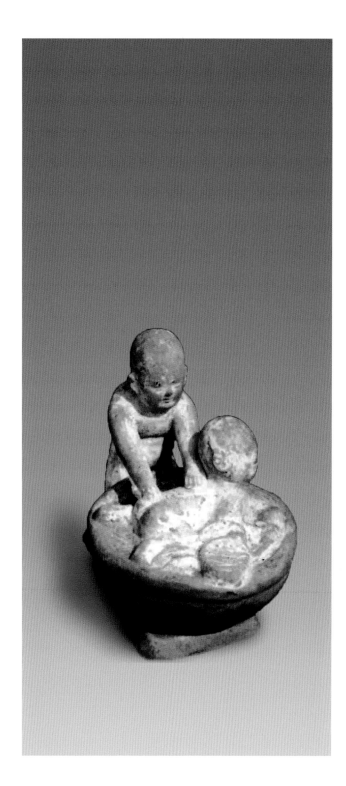

小儿洗澡俑

唐

陶质

盆径 6.5 厘米，通高 8.8 厘米

Tomb Figurine of Bathing Kids

Tang Dynasty

Pottery

Basin Diameter 6.5 cm/ Height 8.8 cm

造型为一小儿站在盆外为爬在盆中的小儿洗澡，生动可爱。西安市出土。

陕西省西安市唐代艺术博物馆藏

This is a vivid figurine of one kid standing outside the basin bathing the baby crawling inside. It was excavated in Xi'an, Shaanxi Province.

Preserved in Xi'an Tang Dynasty Art Museum, Shaanxi Province

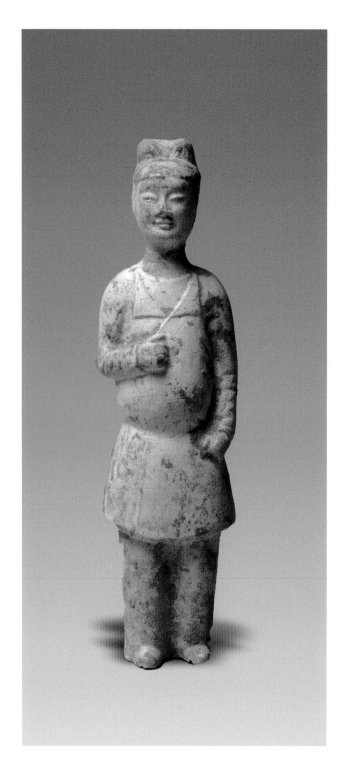

陶侍俑

唐

高 22.5 厘米

Pottery Figurine of a Servant

Tang Dynasty

Height 22.5 cm

头梳双髻，面相丰腴，细眉小口，面露微笑，细小颈，着翻领外衣，束腰，下摆作喇叭形外撇。右手握拳置于胸前，左手握拳贴体下垂。

南京夫子庙展览馆藏

The smiling servant wears double buns. She has a plump face, slim browns, a small mouth, and a slender neck. She wears a garment with an over-turned collar and a tight waist; and the lower hem of the garment flares out. Her right fist clenches in front of her chest while her left fist clenches down her body naturally.
Preserved in the Museum of Confucius Temple in Nanjing

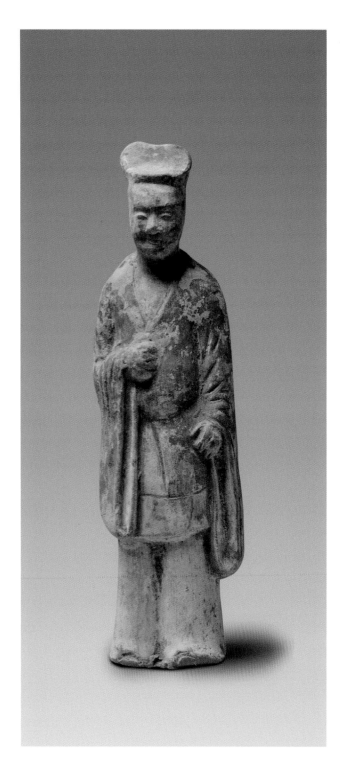

陶侍俑

唐

陶质

高 18.5 厘米

Pottery Figurine of a Servant

Tang Dynasty

Pottery

Height 18.5 cm

戴扇形帽，面相丰颐，着交领大衣，右衽，涂
有彩绘。右手置于胸前，左手贴体下垂。

南京夫子庙展览馆藏

The male servant has a plump face with a fan-
shaped cap. Color painted, the figurine wears
a crossed collar coat with right lapel. His right
hand poses in front of his chest and his left hand
hangs down his body naturally.
Preserved in the Museum of Confucius Temple
in Nanjing

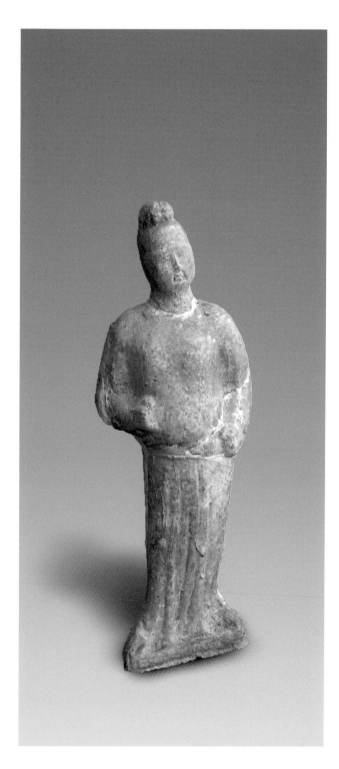

陶仕俑

唐

陶质

高 24 厘米，重 500 克

Pottery Figurine of an Official

Tang Dynasty

Pottery

Height 24 cm/ Weight 500 g

立俑。明器。有残。陕西省咸阳市征集。

陕西医史博物馆藏

Imperfect, the figurine is a funerary object. It
was collected by Xianyang City of Shaanxi
Province.

Preserved in Shaanxi Museum of Medical History

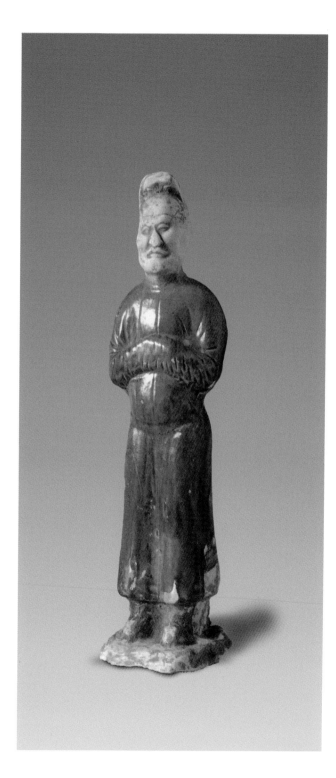

黄釉男仕俑

唐

陶质

高 26.5 厘米

Yellow Glazed Male Official Figurine

Tang Dynasty

Pottery

Height 26.5 cm

头裹巾帽，双手拱于胸前而立，身施黄釉，头、脸、脚均露胎。胎为微微闪红的细泥，较疏松。

郭志强藏

Covered with yellow glaze, the clay figurine is about a male official with headwear. He salutes in a traditional Chinese manner: cupping one hand in the other before chest. The green ware of his head, face and feet are all exposed. The green ware is a kind of fine clay, loosen and lightening.

Collected by Guo Zhiqiang

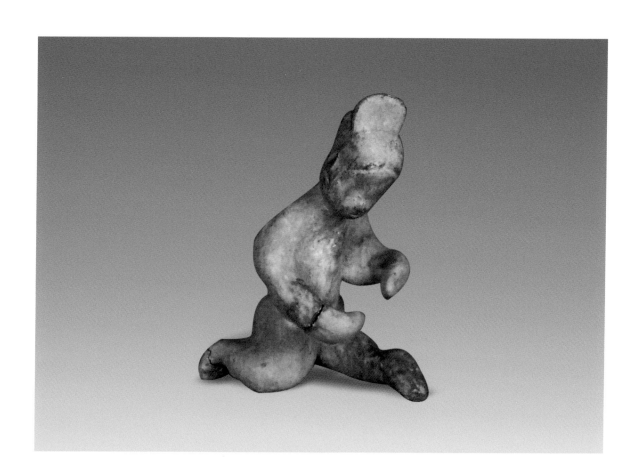

陶俑

唐

陶质

宽 4.9 厘米，通高 8.8 厘米

Pottery Figurine

Tang dynasty

Pottery

Width 4.9 cm/ Height 8.8 cm

明器。该藏为浅棕黄色，人物作奔跑状。1955
年入藏。保存基本完好。

中华医学会 / 上海中医药大学医史博物馆藏

The figurine is in the position of running. It is
a funeral object. It is light yellowish brown. It
was collected in the year of 1955 and is still in
good condition.

Preserved in Chinese Medical Association/ Museum
of Chinese Medicine, Shanghai University of
Traditional Chinese Medicine

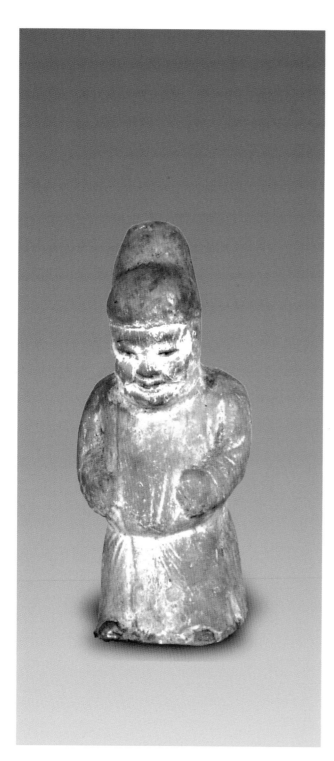

陶人俑

唐

陶质

宽 7.5 厘米，厚 4.8 厘米，通高 15.8 厘米

Pottery Figurine

Tang Dynasty

Pottery

Width 7.5 cm/ Thickness 4.8 cm/ Height 15.8 cm

人像形，明器。该藏为浅棕黄色，人物身着长衫，头戴帽，头略前倾下低。1955 年入藏。保存基本完好。

中华医学会 / 上海中医药大学医史博物馆藏

The figurine is a funeral object. It is in the color of light yellowing brown. The person wears a long gown and a cap with his head lowered forward slightly. It was collected in the year of 1955 and is still in good condition.

Preserved in Chinese Medical Association/Museum of Chinese Medicine, Shanghai University of Traditional Chinese Medicine

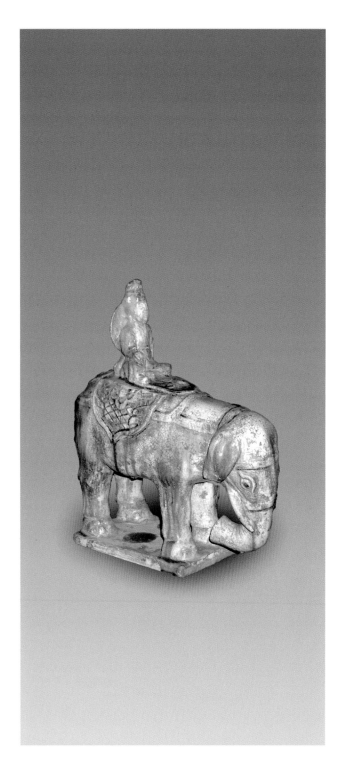

唐三彩坐象俑

唐

陶质

长 28 厘米，宽 11.7 厘米，通高 30.5 厘米，

重 2200 克

象：高 20 厘米

俑：高 10.6 厘米

Elephant-riding Figurine of Tri-colored Pottery

Tang Dynasty

Pottery

Length 28 cm / Width 11.7 cm / Height 30.5 cm /

Weight 2,200 g

Elephant: Height 20 cm

Figurine: Height 10.6 cm

象呈站立状，背上一坐俑，身背斗笠，腿盘曲，

神态悠然自得。工艺品。两耳尖稍残。

陕西医史博物馆藏

The elephant is in the position of standing. A lady is sitting cross-legged lightheartedly on it with a big bamboo hat on her back. It is an artifact. Both tips of the elephant's ears are somewhat damaged.

Preserved in Shaanxi Museum of Medical History

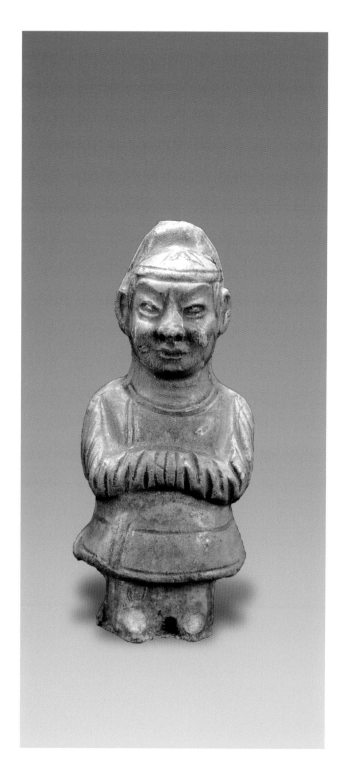

瓷侏儒俑

唐

瓷质

高 18.2 厘米

咸阳市文物保护中心藏

Midget Figurine of Porcelain

Tang Dynasty

Porcelain

Height 18.2 cm

Preserved in the Centre for the Preservation of
Cultural Relics of Xianyang City

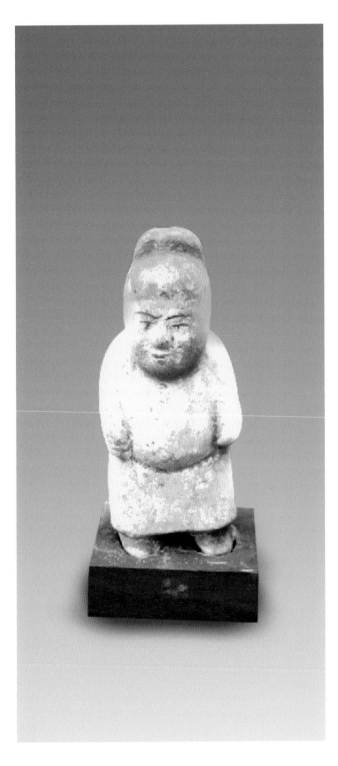

陶质侏儒俑

唐

陶质

宽 3.9 厘米，通高 10.4 厘米，重 145 克

连底座，立式戴帽，束腰，明器。

广东中医药博物馆藏

Midget Figurine of Pottery

Tang Dynasty

Pottery

Width 3.9 cm/ Height 10.4 cm/ Weight 145 g

It is a funeral object with a pedestal. The midget

is standing with a cap and a belt.

Preserved in Guangdong Chinese Medicine Museum

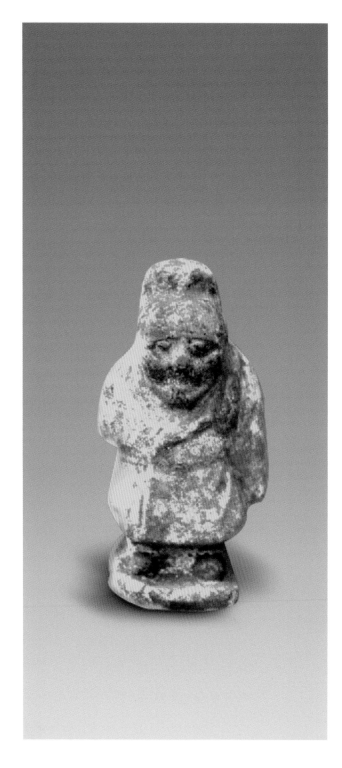

陶质侏儒俑

唐

瓷质

宽 5.4 厘米，通高 10.8 厘米，重 150 克

连底座，立式戴帽，束腰。明器。

广东中医药博物馆藏

Midget Figurine of Porcelain

Tang Dynasty

Porcelain

Width 5.4 cm/ Height 10.8 cm/ Weight 150 g

It is a funeral object with a pedestal. The midget is standing with a turban.

Preserved in Guangdong Chinese Medicine Museum

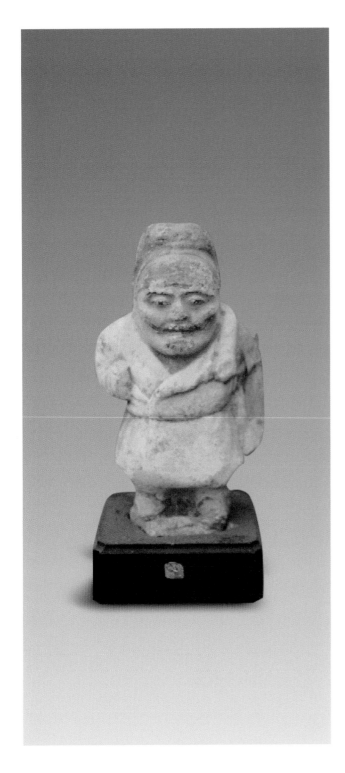

陶质侏儒俑

唐

瓷质

宽 7.9 厘米，通高 12.5 厘米，重 251 克

连底座，立式戴帽，束腰。明器。

广东中医药博物馆藏

Midget Figurine of Pottery

Tang Dynasty

Porcelain

Width 7.9 cm/ Height 12.5 cm/ Weight 251 g

It is a funeral object with a pedestal. The midget

is standing with a cap and a belt.

Preserved in Guangdong Chinese Medicine Museum

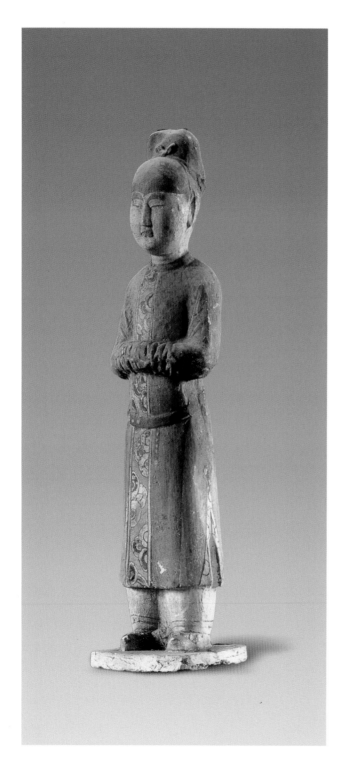

彩绘男装女俑

唐

高 31 厘米

Colored Figurine of a Lady in Man's Wear

Tang Dynasty

Height 31 cm

女俑头戴黑色幞巾，身穿褐色圆领窄袖袍，束腰，穿波斯裤、淡蓝色尖头鞋。

昭陵博物馆藏

With a black silk headscarf, the madam wears a brown long gown with a round collar, narrow sleeves and a waistband. The bottom is a pair of Persian trousers. On her feet is a pair of light blue shoes with a sharp tip.

Preserved in Zhaoling Museum

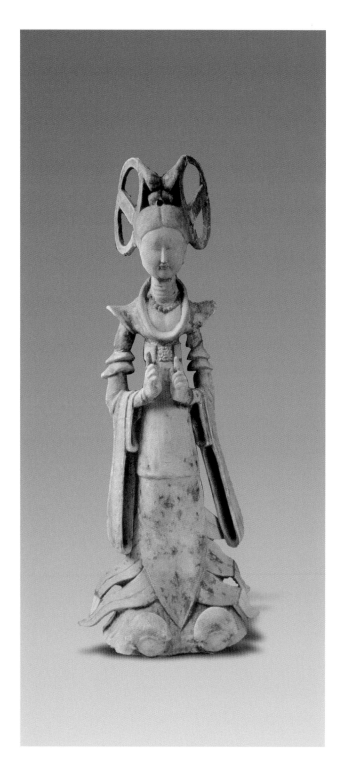

彩绘双环髻女俑

唐

底宽 12.4 厘米，高 37.8 厘米

Colored Figurine of a Lady with Two-ringed Chignons

Tang Dynasty

Base Width 12.4 cm/ Height 37.8 cm

女俑身材颀长，头梳双环髻，脸庞圆润，柳眉细目，颈饰璎珞，削肩纤指。上穿舞袖襦衫，腰系曳地羽裳，脚着云首履，作歌舞状。

长武县博物馆藏

The dancing lady, slim and tall, has a pair of arch eyebrows, two-ringed chignons and a plump face. With slopping shoulders and slender fingers, she wears a necklace of jade and pearls. She wears an short upper garment with dance sleeves. Around her waist are fastened feather clothes which drag to the ground. Her cloud-like shoe-tops are up-turned.

Preserved in Museum of Changwu

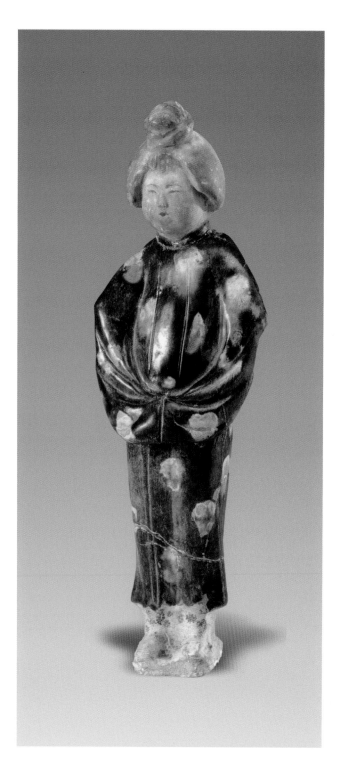

蓝衫女立俑

唐

高 22.5 厘米

Figurine of a Standing Lady in Blue Gown

Tang Dynasty

Height 22.5 cm

女俑身着蓝地白花高领长袍，双手抱于腹前，
体态丰腴。

昭陵博物馆藏

The plump lady wears a long blue gown with
a tall collar. The gown is decorated with white
flowers. Her hands are held in front of her belly.
Preserved in Zhaoling Museum

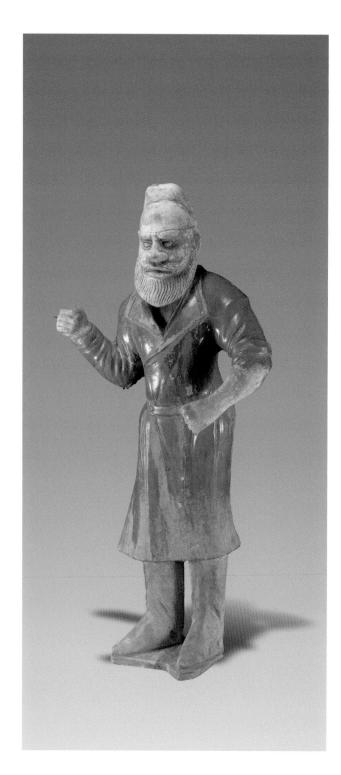

三彩控马男立俑

唐

高 71 厘米

Tri-colored Glazed Figurine of a Standing Horseman

Tang Dynasty

Height 71 cm

此俑表现胡人形象，神情刻画准确细腻，堪称唐塑精品。

故宫博物院藏

The figurine depicts an image of Hu people in Tang Dynasty. The facial expression is made accurate and delicate. It is a competitive product among Tang statues.

Preserved in the Palace Museum

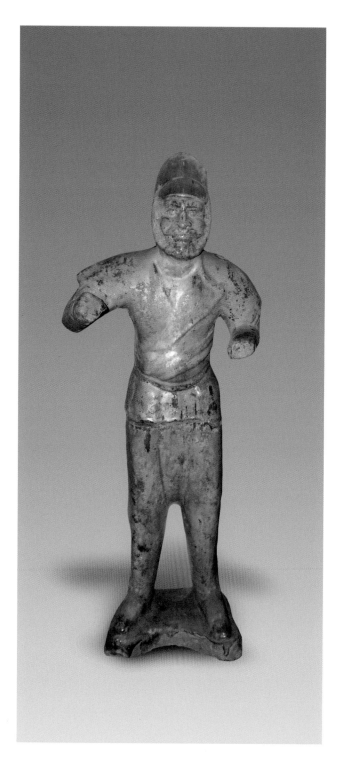

牵驼俑

唐

陶质

高 51 厘米

Pottery Figurine of a Camel Leading Man

Tang Dynasty

Pottery

Height 51 cm

通体绿釉，一波斯男性成年男子站立形象，手势呈牵驼样。明器。稍残有修复。陕西省咸阳市博物馆调拨。

陕西医史博物馆藏

The figurine is covered with green glaze. It is a funeral object. The adult Persian is in the position of standing. He gestures to be leading a camel. It is incomplete but repaired. The figurine was allocated from the Xianyang Museum, Shaanxi.

Preserved in Shaanxi Museum of Medical History

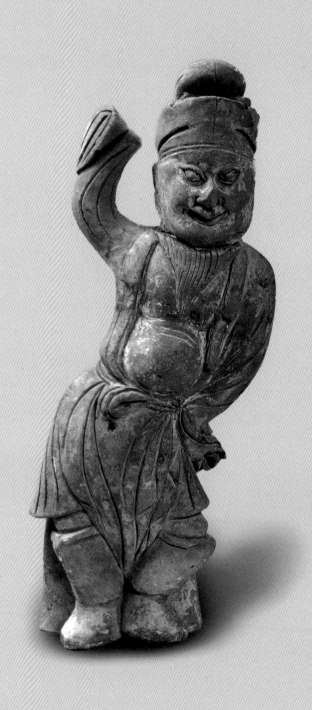

男舞俑

南唐

泥质灰陶质

高 46 厘米

头戴幞头，颌下长须飘髯，身着窄袖长袍，腰间束带，袒胸露腹，足蹬靴，扬手扭腰，作舞蹈状。通体施白、红粉。该俑是当时宫廷乐舞侍从的具体写照，形象生动。江宁祖堂山南唐李昇钦陵出土。

南京博物院藏

Figurine of a Male Dancer

Southern Tang Dynasty

Grey Clay Pottery

Height 46 cm

With a kerchief on the head, long beards and sideburns around the chin, the bare-chested figurine dresses in a narrow-sleeved robe with a belt worn at the waist and boots on the feet. He is waving his hands and twisting his waist as if dancing. The whole figurine is in white and reddish-pink. It vividly portrays the specific image of the dancing attendants at the royal court back then. It was excavated from the tomb of Li Bianqin of the Southern Tang Dynasty on Zu Tang Mountain, Jiangning, Jiangsu Province.

Preserved in Nanjing Museum

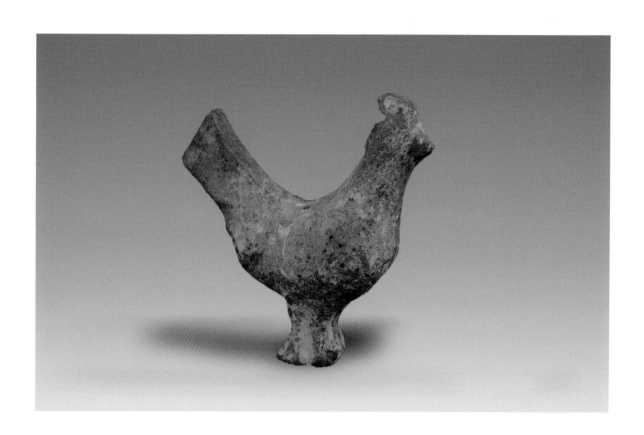

陶鸡

唐

红陶质

通高 11.5 厘米，重 150 克

鸡形，红陶色。明器。艺术品。嘴部稍残。

陕西医史博物馆藏

Pottery Chicken

Tang Dynasty

Red Pottery

Height 11.5 cm/ Weight 150 g

The chicken is in the color of red pottery. It is a funeral and art ware. The chicken's beak is broken.

Preserved in Shaanxi Museum of Medical History

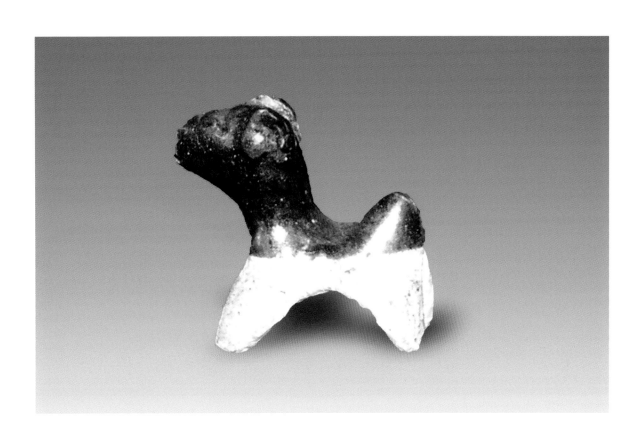

Porcelain Puppy

Tang Dynasty

Porcelain

Long Diameter 4 cm/ Bottom Diameter 3 cm/
Height 3.5 cm/ Weight 40 g

The dog's body is black-glazed but all the four feet
bare. As a toy, it is lively shaped. It is intact and
undamaged. It was collected from Qindu District of
Xianyang City, Shaanxi Province.

Preserved in Shaanxi Museum of Medical History

小瓷狗

唐

瓷质

长口径 4 厘米，底径 3 厘米，通高 3.5 厘米，重
40 克

小狗身上为黑釉，四足无釉，造型生动。玩具，
完整无损，陕西省咸阳市秦都区征集。

陕西医史博物馆藏

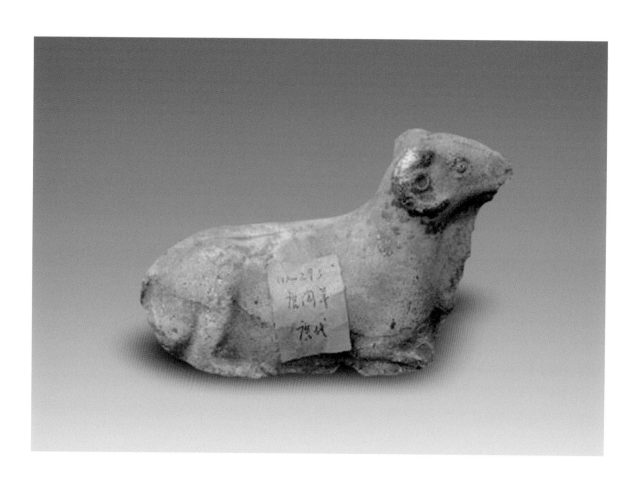

陶羊

唐

瓷质

长 13.1 厘米，宽 5 厘米，通高 7.65 厘米，重 235 克

卧式绵羊，昂首。随葬品。

广东中医药博物馆藏

Pottery Sheep

Tang Dynasty

Porcelain

Long 13.1 cm/ Width 5 cm/ Height 7.65 cm/
Weight 235 g

The sheep is crouching and holding its head high. It
is a burial object.

Preserved in Guangdong Chinese Medicine Museum

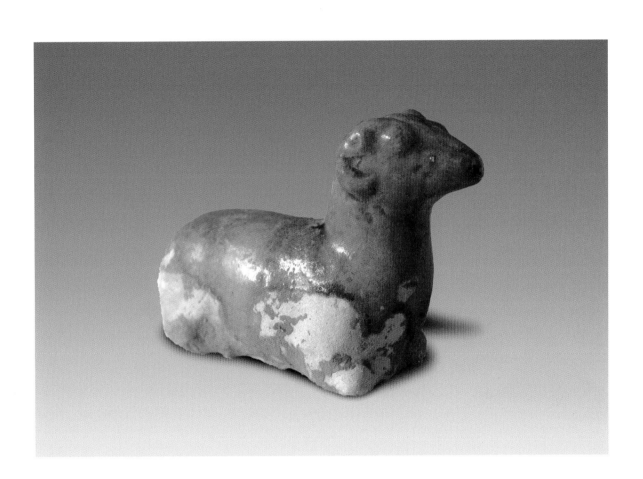

黄釉羊

唐

羊为卧式，伸颈，昂首。全身施黄釉，釉质莹润，釉开细纹片，胎为闪淡红色细泥白胎，胎质较松。唐代明器。

叶耀藏

Yellow Glazed Sheep

Tang Dynasty

The sheep is lying down with stretched neck and raised head. It is glazed in yellow. The glaze is lustrous and transparent with fine lines. The green ware is made of fine white earth with loosen nature. It is a burial object of Tang Dynasty.

Collected by Yeyao

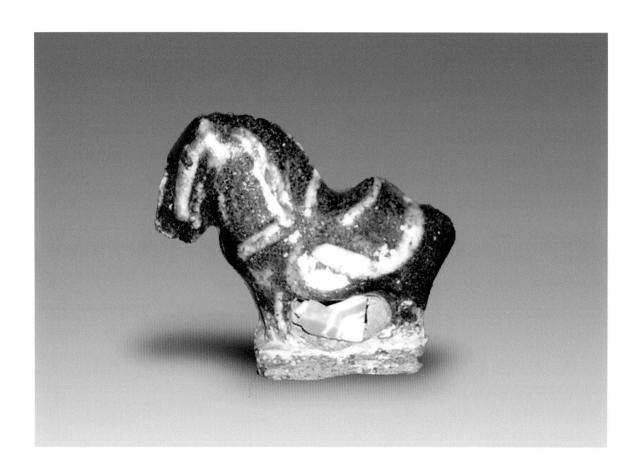

小瓷马

唐

瓷质

长口径 4.3 厘米，底径 2.5 厘米，通高 4 厘米，重 50 克

Porcelain Pony

Tang Dynasty

Porcelain

Long Diameter 4.3 cm/ Bottom Diameter 2.5 cm/ Height 4 cm/ Weight 50 g

一立马，方形底座，马背弯曲，黑釉身上有白
斑纹。瓷塑玩具。完整无损。陕西省咸阳市秦
都区征集。

陕西医史博物馆藏

The horse is standing on a quadrate base. Its
back bends and white strips disperse in the
black glaze. As a porcelain toy, it is intact
and undamaged. It was collected from Qindu
District of Xianyang City of Shaanxi Province.
Preserved in Shaanxi Museum of Medical History

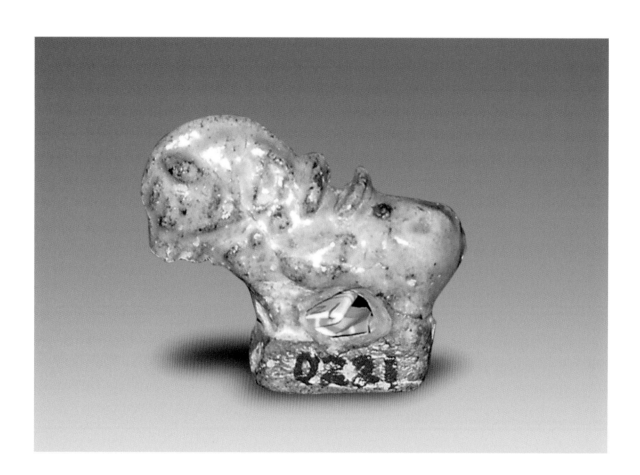

小瓷马

唐

瓷质

长口径 5 厘米，底径 2.5 厘米，通高 4.1 厘米，重 50 克

Porcelain Pony

Tang Dynasty

Porcelain

Long Diameter 5 cm/ Bottom Diameter 2.5 cm/ Height 4.1 cm/ Weight 50 g

一立马，马背弯曲，方形底座，米色釉。瓷塑，
玩具，嘴部有残，陕西省咸阳市秦都区征集。

陕西医史博物馆藏

The horse stands on a rectangular base with
bending back. As a porcelain toy, it wears cream
color glaze. Its mouth is fragmentary. It was
collected from Qindu District of Xianyang City
of Shaanxi Province.

Preserved in Shaanxi Museum of Medical History

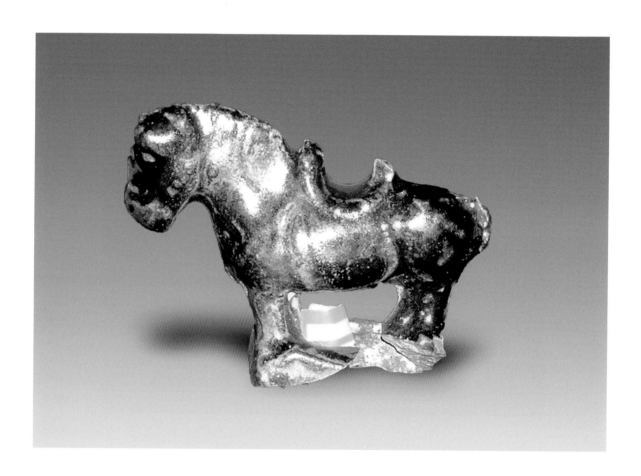

小瓷马

唐

瓷质

长口径 7 厘米，底径 3.5 厘米，通高 5.6 厘米，重 50 克

Porcelain Pony

Tang Dynasty

Porcelain

Long Diameter 7 cm/ Bottom Diameter 3.5 cm/ Height 5.6 cm/ Weight 50 g

一立马，方形底座，马背弯曲，黑釉。瓷塑，
玩具。底座有残。陕西省咸阳市秦都区征集。

陕西医史博物馆藏

The horse wears black glaze and stands on
a rectangular base with bending back. It is a
porcelain toy and the base is incomplete. It was
collected from Qindu District of Xianyang City
of Shaanxi Province.
Preserved in Shaanxi Museum of Medical History

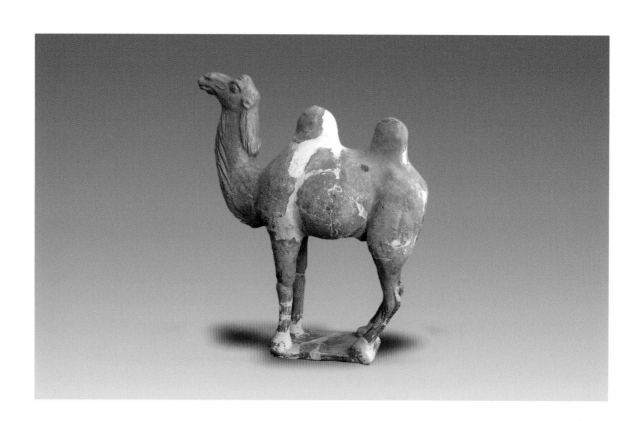

陶骆驼

唐

陶质

通高 38.5 厘米，重 3150 克

底座：长 14.6 厘米，宽 9.5 厘米

Pottery Camel

Tang dynasty

Pottery

Height 38.5 cm/ Weight 3,150 g

Base: Length 14.6 cm/ Width 9.5 cm

昂首，双峰驼，腹空。明器。有残。陕西省咸
阳市征集。

陕西医史博物馆藏

The pottery camel has double humps with a
raising head and an empty belly. It is a funerary
ware and incomplete. It was collected from
Xianyang of Shaanxi Province.

Preserved in Shaanxi Museum of Medical History

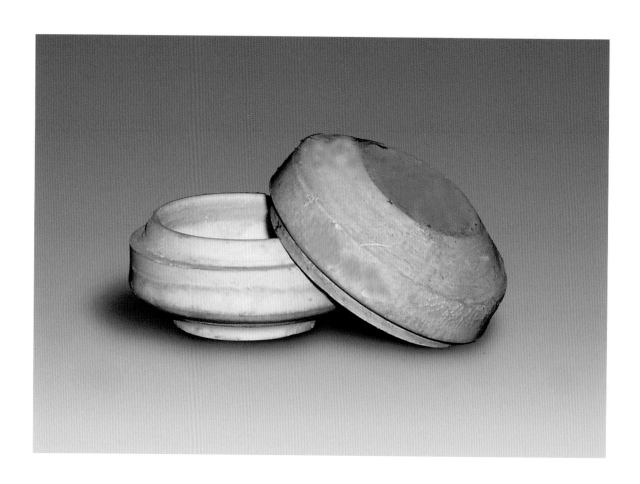

瓷盒

唐

瓷质

口径 5 厘米，底径 3 厘米，通高 4 厘米，重 100 克

Porcelain Box

Tang Dynasty

Porcelain

Mouth Diameter 5 cm/ Bottom Diameter 3 cm/ Height 4 cm/ Weight 100 g

子母口，直腹，圈足，白瓷无纹饰。盛贮器。
完整无损。陕西省西安市征集。

陕西医史博物馆藏

The box, glazed white with no decoration on the
surface, has a double lip mouth buckled with a
lid, straight walls and a ring foot. This reservoir
vessel, collected in Xi'an, is completely intact.
Preserved in Shaanxi Museum of Medical History

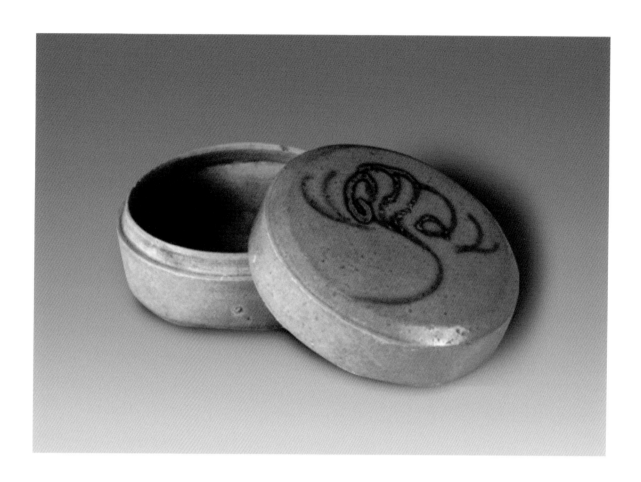

青釉绿彩油盒

唐

瓷质

口径 10.1 厘米，高 5.5 厘米

Celadon Powder Box with Paintings in Green

Tang Dynasty

Porcelain

Mouth Diameter 10.1 cm/ Height 5.5 cm

盒为扁圆形，盖与盒成子母口套合，平底。盖面绘绿彩卷云纹，线条随意流畅。胎色灰白，质粗疏。内外满施釉，釉色青翠光亮。此盒为贮存化妆品的容器，出土的同类瓷盒盖面上有书"油合"铭文的。1963年扬州平山乡朱塘村出土。

扬州博物馆藏

The box is oblate-shaped with a flat bottom and a box cover which can be buckled with the box body. On the lid is painted a smoothly and naturally outlined pattern of scrolled clouds in green. With the crude body in greyish-white, the interior and exterior of the box are fully glazed light green. This vessel was used to keep cosmetics, with an inscription "You He" on the lid. It was excavated in Zhutang Village of Pingshan Township in Yangzhou, Jiangsu Province, in 1963.

Preserved in Yangzhou Museum

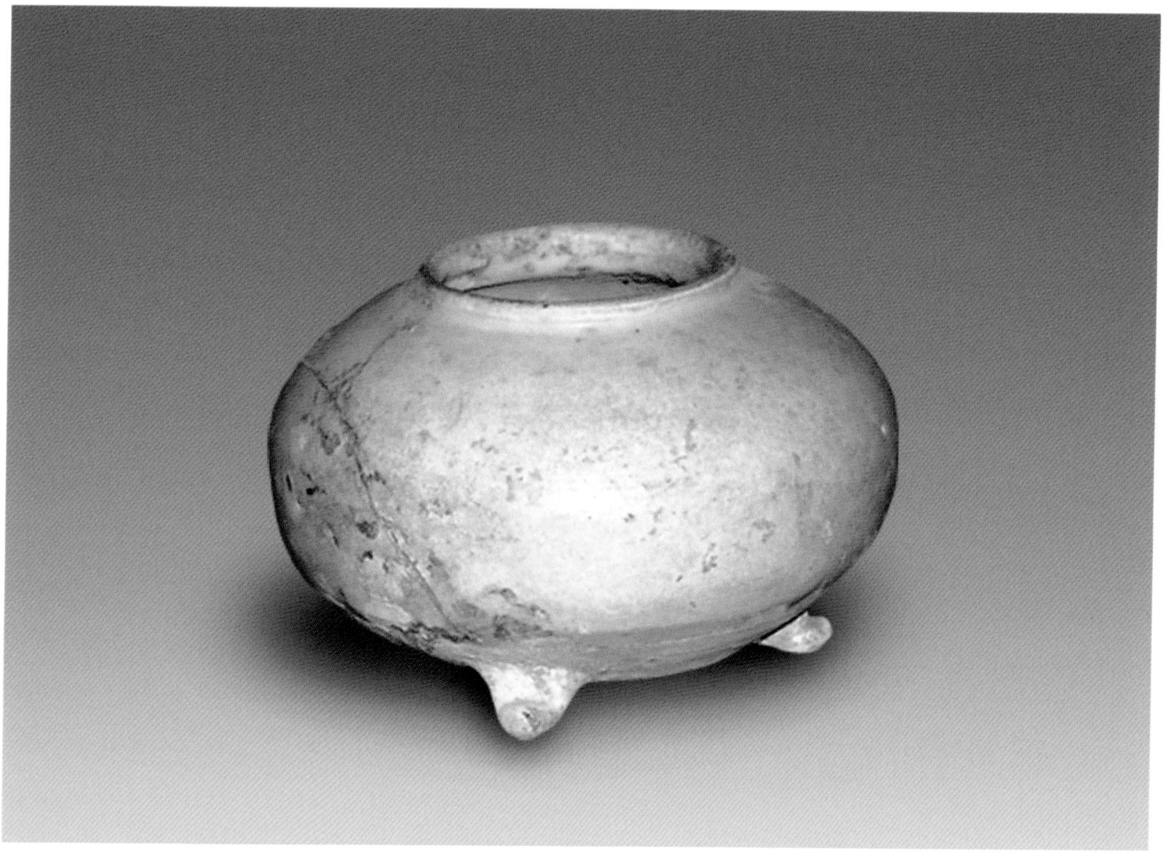

白瓷唾盂

唐

瓷质

口径 3.7 厘米，底径 4.4 厘米，高 4.7 厘米，重 100 克

White Porcelain Spittoon

Tang Dynasty

Porcelain

Mouth Diameter 3.7 cm/ Bottom Diameter 4.4 cm/ Height 4.7 cm/ Weight 100 g

圆唇，斜肩，直腹，平底，底有三小足，白釉

泛青。卫生器具。腹有裂痕。2001 年 9 月入藏。

陕西省西安市古玩市场征集。

陕西医史博物馆藏

The spittoon has a round lip, drooping

shoulders, straight walls and a flat bottom with

three short legs. It is covered with bluish-white

glaze with crackles on the stomach. This piece

of sanitary ware was collected in Xi'an antique

market in Shaanxi Province in September 2001.

Preserved in Shaanxi Museum of Medical History

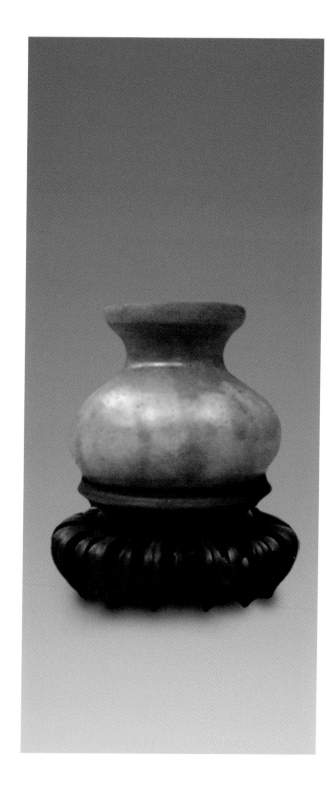

唾盂

唐

瓷质

口径 8.9 厘米，腹径 13.2 厘米，通高 10.5 厘米

Spittoon

Tang Dynasty

Porcelain

Mouth 8.9 cm/ Belly Diameter 13.2 cm/ Height

10.5 cm

该藏通身施青黄色釉，平底，假圈足，喇叭口，

工艺一般。盂形，为卫生用具。1957 年入藏。

保存基本完好。

中华医学会 / 上海中医药大学医史博物馆藏

This cuspidor-shaped spittoon, a sanitary utensil,

is coated with greenish yellow glaze. It has a

wide trumpet-shaped mouth and a flat bottom in

the form of a ring foot. The craftsmanship is of

average level. It was collected in the year 1957

and is well preserved.

Preserved in Chinese Medical Association/Museum

of Chinese Medicine, Shanghai University of

Traditional Chinese Medicine

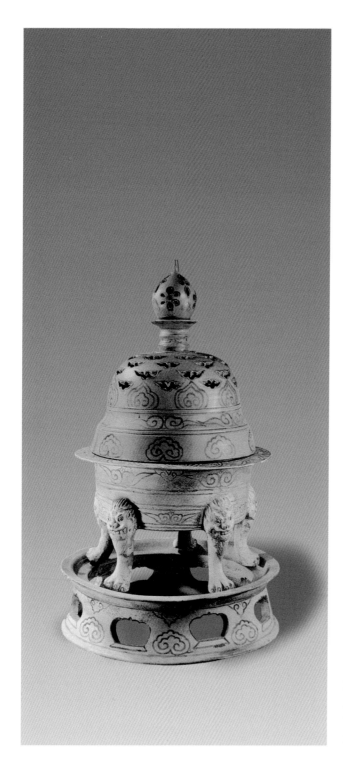

越窑褐彩云纹五足炉

唐

瓷质

口径 36.5 厘米，底径 41 厘米，通高 66 厘米

Five-footed Incense Burner with Brown Cloud Design, Yue Kiln

Tang Dynasty

Porcelain

Mouth Diameter 36.5 cm/ Bottom Diameter 41 cm/

Height 66 cm

器由盖、炉和座三部分组成。1980 年浙江临

安唐天复元年（901）水邱氏墓出土。

临安市文物管理委员会藏

This ware is composed of three parts: lid,
incense burner and bottom. It was excavated
from the tomb of Ms. Shuiqiu who died in
the 1st year (A.D. 901) of Tianfu Reign, Tang
Dynasty, in Lin'an, Zhejiang Province, in the
year 1980.

Preserved in the Department of Cultural Relics
Conservation of Lin'an

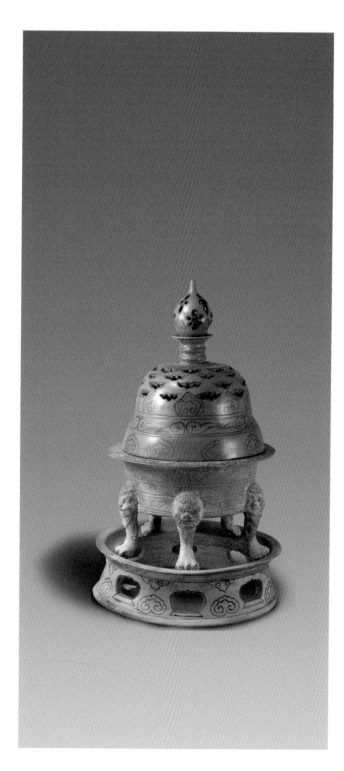

褐彩如意云纹青瓷熏炉

唐

瓷质

高 66 厘米

Celadon Incense Burner Painted with Brown Ruyi-shaped Cloud Motif

Tang Dynasty

Porcelain

Height 66 cm

全器由盖、炉、座三部分组成，通体施青釉，由于烧成气氛不同，盖与炉、座釉色不同。盖部釉呈青黄色，炉和座因窑温较低等原因，未能达到良好的烧成效果。盖、炉、座均绘釉下褐彩如意状云纹。

临安市文物馆藏

The entirely glazed ware is composed of three parts: lid, censer and base, the glaze colours of which are different on account of different firing atmosphere. The lid is glazed greenish yellow, but the censer as well as the base failed to reach the best quality, due to the low temperature in the kiln during the firing process. All three parts are decorated with underglaze brown Ruyi-shaped cloud motifs.

Preserved in Lin'an Museum of Cultural Relics

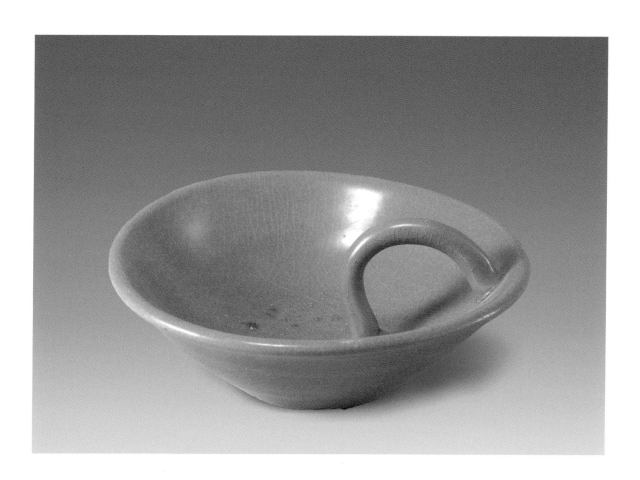

灯

唐

瓷质

口径 13 厘米，高 5.3 厘米

Lamp

Tang Dynasty

Porcelain

Mouth Diameter 13 cm/ Height 5.3 cm

敞口，斜直腹，小平底略上凹弧。内有一环，

青釉泛黄，外底无釉，有 6 个泥点痕。

浙江省文物考古研究所藏

The lamp has a flared mouth, sloping walls and
a slightly concave base. With a ring attached
to the interior wall, the lamp is covered with
yellowish celadon, while the exterior bottom is
unglazed, on which can be seen six mud marks.
Preserved in Institute of Cultural Relics and
Archaeology of Zhejiang Province

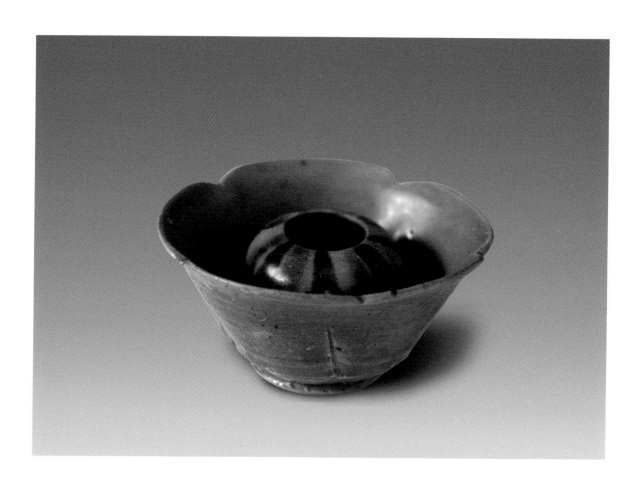

长沙铜官窑青釉灯盏

唐

瓷质

口径 11.5 厘米，底径 5 厘米，高 4.5 厘米

Celadon Oil Lamp, Changsha Tongguan Kiln

Tang Dynasty

Porcelain

Mouth Diameter 11.5 cm/ Bottom Diameter 5 cm/ Height 4.5 cm

灯托为五花瓣口碗形，托内为圆形小水注，托施青黄色釉，盏深青黄釉加绘褐彩斑纹釉。该造型有其科学性，利于防风防火灾，应属于晚唐作品。

吴德蔚藏

The lamp saucer is in the shape of a bowl with five-lobed mouth rim. The saucer, with a small cylindrical water jet inside, is coated with greenish-yellow glaze, while the lamp is covered with dark greenish-yellow glaze painted with brown dappled glaze. It was designed in such a way as to be wind-proof and fire-proof. This piece belongs to the late Tang Dynasty ware.

Collected by Wu Dewei

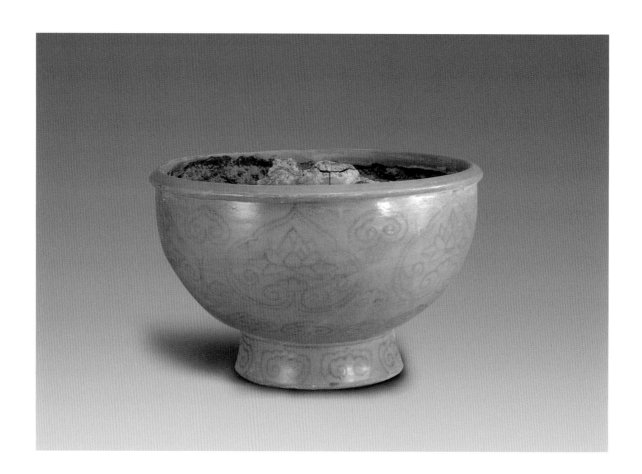

褐彩青瓷油灯

唐

瓷质

口径 37.2 厘米，底径 19.5 厘米，高 24.4 厘米

Celadon Oil Lamp with Brown Paintings

Tang Dynasty

Porcelain

Mouth Diameter 37.2 cm/ Bottom Diameter 19.5 cm/ Height 24.4 cm

器形较大，通体青釉，呈青黄色，有冰裂纹。

釉下彩绘褐彩如意云纹。

临安市文物馆藏

This lamp has a quite large body entirely
covered by greenish-yellow celadon with ice
crackles and decorated with underglaze brown
Ruyi-shaped cloud motifs.

Preserved in Lin'an Museum of Cultural Relics

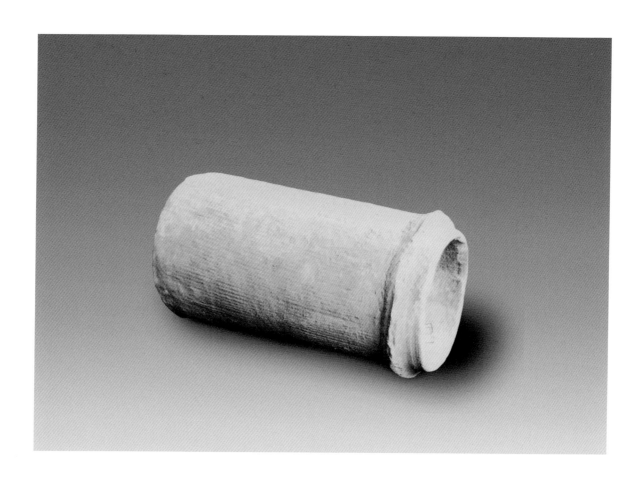

圆形陶下水道

唐

陶质

长 33.5 厘米，内口径 12 厘米，外口径 17.5 厘米

Round Sewer Pipe

Tang Dynasty

Pottery

Length 33.5 cm/ Inner Diameter 12 cm/ Outer Diameter 17.5 cm

两端有接合之子母口，通身绳纹。这种水道在
相互连接上较秦汉水道有很大进步。西安市北
郊大明宫遗址出土。

陕西医史博物馆藏

The sewer pipe has a buckle design at both
ends for connection with cord patterns incised
on the surface. Compared with the sewer pipes
in the Qin and Han Dynasties, this one is more
advanced in its connection design. It was
excavated from Da Ming Palace Ruins of the
Tang Dynasty, located in the northern suburbs
of Xi'an, Shaanxi Province.

Preserved in Shaanxi Museum of Medical History

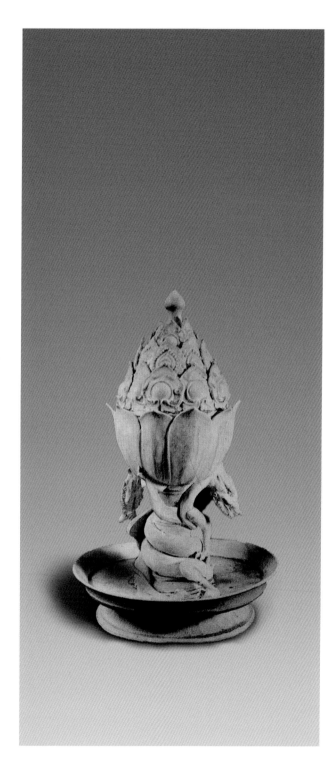

蟠龙博山炉

唐

白瓷质

高 38 厘米

Bo Shan Censer with Coiling Dragon Design

Tang Dynasty

White Porcelain

Height 38 cm

炉身呈青铜器。由炉座、炉盘、炉盖三部分组成。

炉座圈足，有三条蟠龙盘旋，龙头托住炉盘；

炉身似盛开的荷花；炉盖似高低起伏的山峦。

日本大和文华馆藏

The bronze censer is composed of a base, a saucer and a lid. On the ring-foot base, three curled-up dragons are coiled together to hold the saucer. The body of the censer looks like a blossoming lotus, while the lid is in the shape of rolling hills.

Preserved in Museum Yamato Bunkakan in Japan

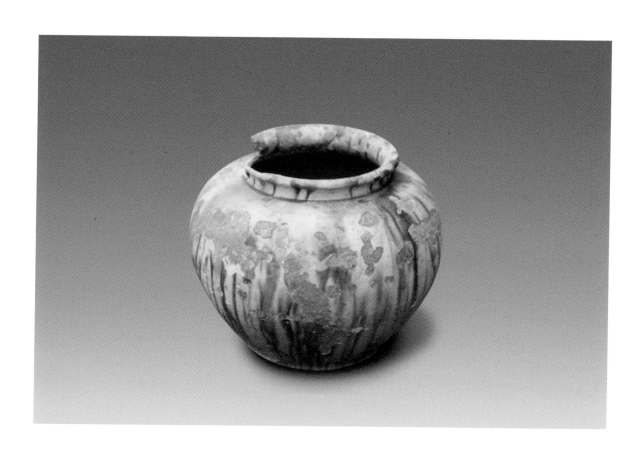

绿釉陶罐

唐

陶质

外口径 13.2 厘米，腹径 21.7 厘米，底径 13.3 厘米，

通高 17 厘米，腹深 16.3 厘米，重 1450 克

敞口，鼓腹，平底。盛物容器。

广东中医药博物馆藏

Green-glazed Pottery Jar

Tang Dynasty

Pottery

Outer Mouth Diameter 13.2 cm/ Belly Diameter

21.7 cm/ Bottom Diameter 13.3 cm/ Height 17 cm/

Depth 16.3 cm/ Weight 1,450 g

This bottle has a flared mouth, a melon-shaped belly

and a flat bottom. It was utilized as a container.

Preserved in Guangdong Chinese Medicine Museum

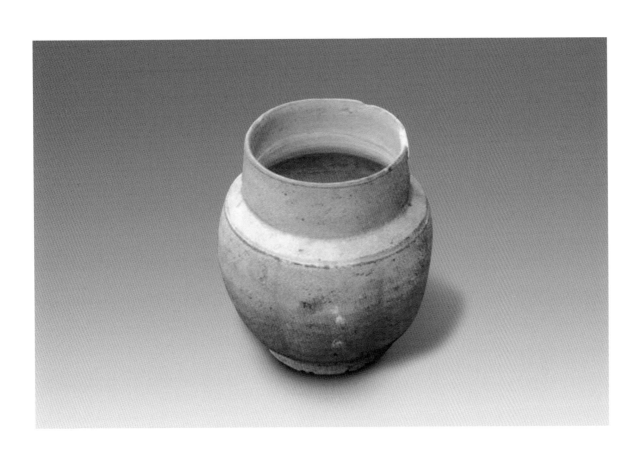

青釉陶罐

五代

陶质

外口径 8.3 厘米，腹径 11.7 厘米，底径 7.6 厘米，

通高 13.2 厘米，腹深 15.3 厘米

直口，粗颈，圆腹，圈足，盛物容器。

广东中医药博物馆藏

Celadon-glazed Pottery Jar

Five Dynasties

Pottery

Outer Mouth Diameter 8.3 cm/ Belly Diameter

11.7 cm/ Bottom Diameter 7.6 cm/ Height 13.2 cm/

Depth 15.3 cm

This jar has a straight mouth, a broad neck, a round

belly and a ring foot. It was used as a container.

Preserved in Guangdong Chinese Medicine Museum

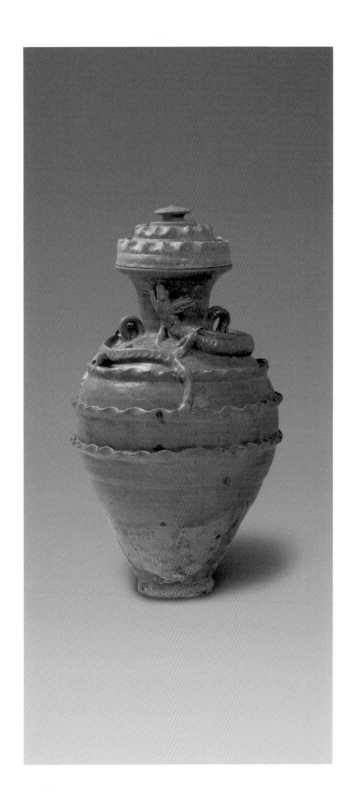

青釉塑龙纹瓷盖瓶

唐—五代

瓷质

口径18厘米，腹径35.6厘米，底径11.6厘米，

高56.6厘米

Covered Celadon Vase with Carved Dragon Patterns

Tang Dynasty–the Five Dynasties

Porcelain

Mouth Diameter 18 cm/ Belly Diameter 35.6 cm/

Bottom Diameter 11.6 cm/ Height 56.6 cm

敛口，束颈，溜肩，鼓腹，渐收至底，圈足稍外撇。灰白胎，施青釉不到底。帽形瓶盖，尖顶钮，口饰刻画流云纹，子母瓶口，肩部堆塑对称复系。瓶身上部堆塑二条盘龙，龙身细长满鳞。瓶腹部堆塑水波纹并刻画流云纹。此瓶形体高大，为越窑优秀作品。

南京博物院藏

This vase has a contracted mouth and neck, a sloping shoulder, a bulging belly tapering downwards to the bottom, and a ring foot slightly everting outwards. It is celadon-glazed except its lower part and bottom, exposing the greyish white body. The lid is in the shape of a hat with a pointed knob. The mouth of the vase, in snap-in design, is incised with cloud patterns, while its shoulder is decorated with symmetric double rings. Two coiling dragons, whose slender body is fully covered with scales, are moulded on the upper part of the vase. The belly of the vase is embossed with water ripples and incised with cloud patterns. Big in size, the vase is an exquisite example of Yue kiln ware.

Preserved in Nanjing Museum

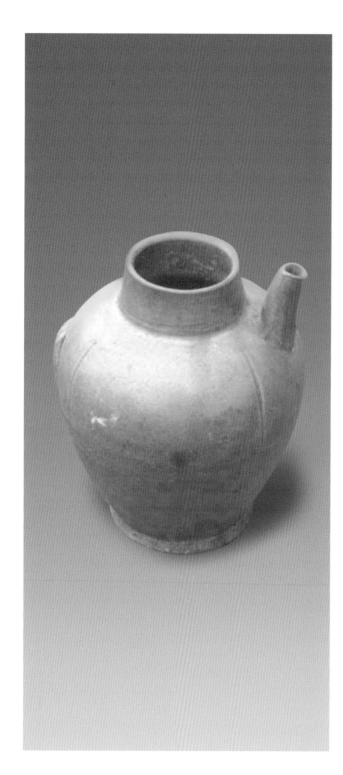

越窑瓷壶

五代

瓷质

外口径 4.9 厘米，腹径 11.2 厘米，底径 7 厘米，

通高 14 厘米，腹深 13 厘米

Porcelain Ewer, Yue Ware

Five Dynasties

Porcelain

Outer Mouth Diameter 4.9 cm/ Diameter 11.2
cm/ Bottom Diameter 7 cm/ Belly Height 14 cm/
Depth 13 cm

平口，鼓腹，腹上丰下敛，无耳，一短流，流垂直向上，平底，底边沿外张。盛酒等液体容器。

广东中医药博物馆藏

This earless ewer, has a flat mouth, a vertical short spout, a swelling belly and a flat bottom. The lower part of the belly tapers downwards, and its bottom rim extends outward. It was used as a liquid vessel.

Preserved in Guangdong Chinese Medicine Museum

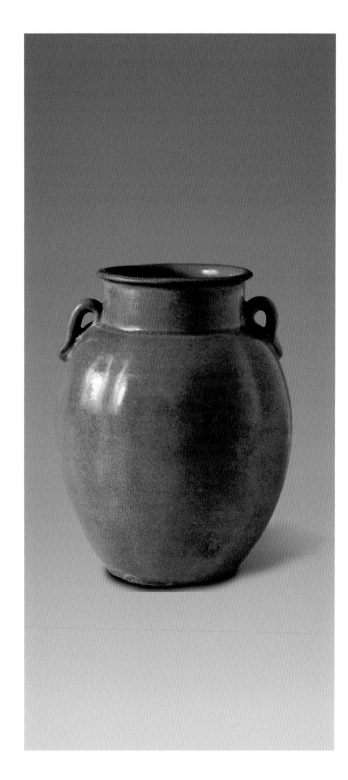

越窑青瓷双系罐

五代

瓷质

口径 6.2 厘米，底径 5.5 厘米，高 11.5 厘米

Celadon Jar with Double rings, Yue Ware

Five Dynasties

Porcelain

Mouth Diameter 6.2 cm/ Bottom Diameter 5.5 cm/

Height 11.5 cm

短直颈，口缘外卷，瓜棱式丰腹，卧足。肩颈之间设对称的圆状式系。全身施青釉，略带黄色。釉细润，开细小纹片。足无釉露灰色胎，外表呈浅酱色，有六个支烧痕迹。五代越窑器代表作品。

李毓麟藏

The jar has a short straight neck, an everted mouth-rim, a melon-shaped belly and a horizontal foot with two symmetrical ears between the neck and the shoulder. Its whole body is coated with exquisite and mellow celadon glaze shining slightly yellowish tints with small crackles. The bottom of the jar is unglazed, revealing its grey body, and shows light reddish brown in colour. Six burning marks can be seen on the bottom. The jar is a representative work of Yue kiln of the Five Dynasties.

Collected by Li Yulin

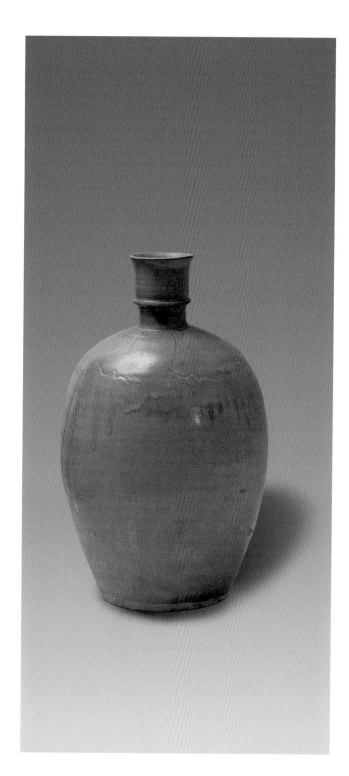

青釉莲花纹瓷梅瓶

五代

瓷质

口径 7 厘米，底径 14.5 厘米，高 37 厘米

Celadon Prunus Vase with Lotus Pattern

Five Dynasties

Porcelain

Mouth Diameter 7 cm/ Bottom Diameter 14.5 cm/

Height 37 cm

侈口，细颈，圆腹。肩部饰一周刻画莲瓣荷叶纹，

手法随意，通体施淡青釉，厚薄不均，有积釉痕。

底无釉露灰白胎，有烧制痕迹。系越窑青瓷。

南京博物院藏

The vase is characterized with a flared mouth,
a narrow neck and a round belly. Around its
shoulder are patterns of lotus petals and leaves
incised in a free style. The vase is unevenly
glazed with light celadon, and marks of
accumulated glaze can be seen. Its unglazed
bottom reveals its grey-white body and signs of
firing. It belongs to celadon ware from Yue kiln.
Preserved in Nanjing Museum

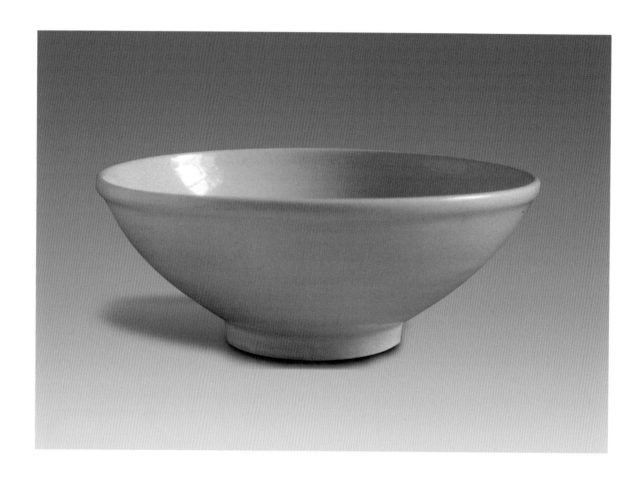

定窑白釉碗

五代

瓷质

口径 18.3 厘米，高 7 厘米

White-glazed Bowl, Ding Ware

Five Dynasties

Porcelain

Mouth Diameter 18.3 cm/ Height 7 cm

敞口，卷唇，弧形腹，浅圈足。里外施白釉，釉稍冷青色，不匀处有泪痕，属早期定窑产品。定窑在河北省曲阳涧磁村及东西燕川村，古属定州，因此得名。创烧于唐，极盛于北宋及金，停烧于元代。

卢晓辉藏

This bowl has a wide mouth with a rolled rim, an arc-shaped belly, and a short ring foot. The interior and exterior are white-glazed with a hint of cold cyan. Where glaze coagulated, glaze drips like "tear stains" can be seen. The bowl is an example of the early Ding ware. Ding kiln is located at Jianci Village，East Yanchuan Village and West Yanchuan Village of Quyang in Hebei Province, which belonged to Dingzhou in ancient times. Ding kiln was named after that. Ding kiln started its manufacture in the Tang Dynasty, and became extremely popular in the Northern Song Dynasty and the Jin Dynasty. It was closed in the Yuan Dynasty.

Collected by Lu Xiaohui

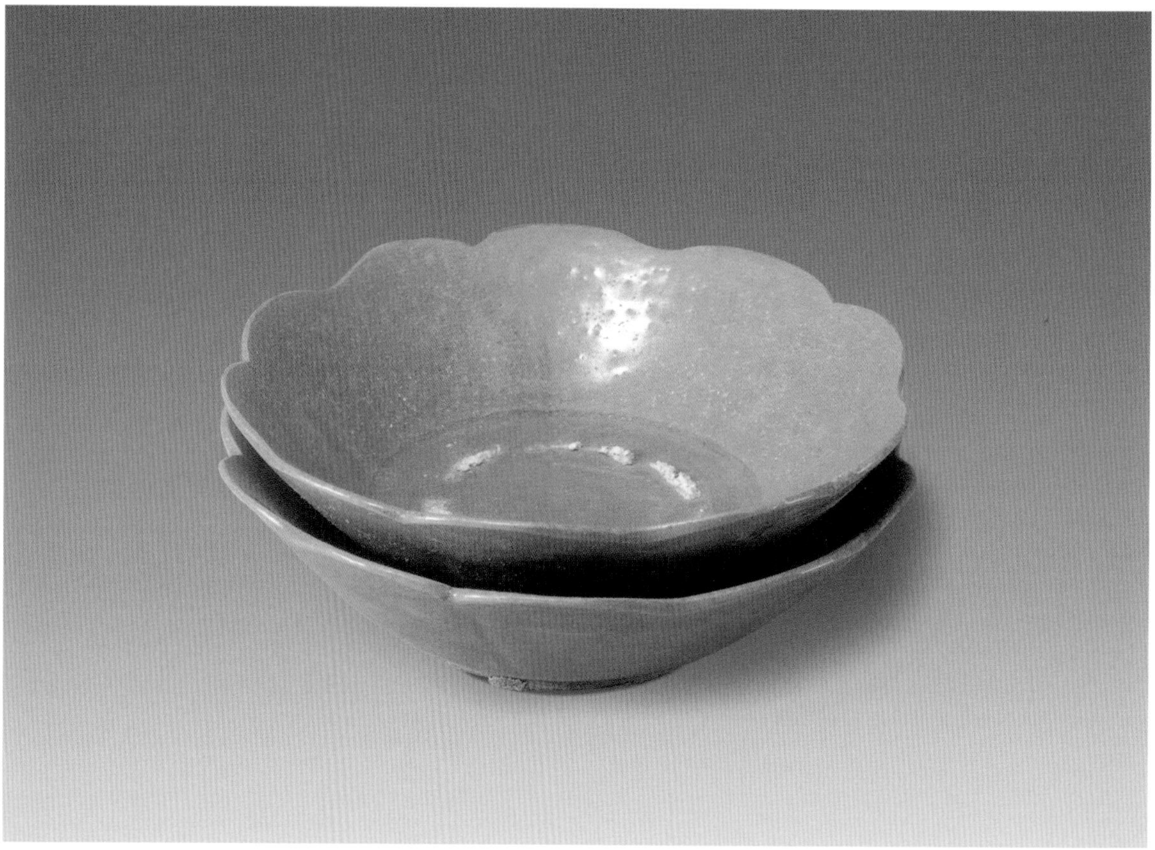

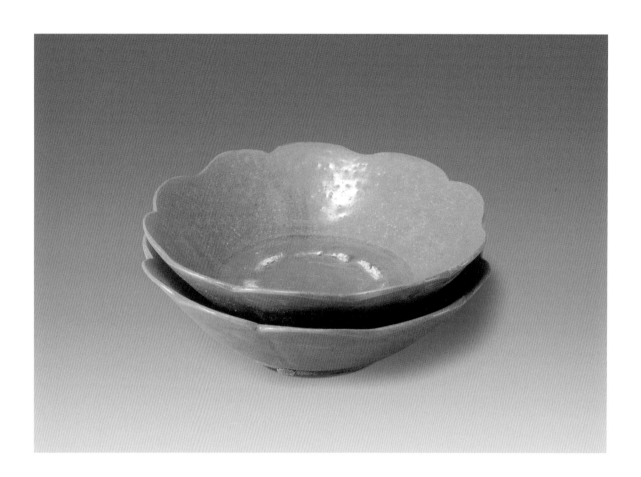

碟

五代

瓷质

口径 14 厘米，高 4.6 厘米

Plate

Five Dynasties

Porcelain

Mouth Diameter 14 cm/ Height 4.6 cm

整器犹如荷花，腹壁斜直，内底宽平，圈足较

矮小。满青釉泛黄，足刮釉。临安康陵所出碟

与此同。1998 年慈溪市寺龙口窑址出土。

浙江省文物考古研究所藏

The plate resembles a lotus, with a sloping wall,
a wide and flat interior bottom and a short ring
foot. The body is covered with yellowish-green
glaze, except its foot rim. The plate is similar to
the one unearthed in Kangling of Lin'an. It was
unearthed from Silongkou kiln site of Cixi City,
Zhejiang Province, in the year 1998.
Preserved in Institute of Cultural Relics and
Archaeology of Zhejiang Province

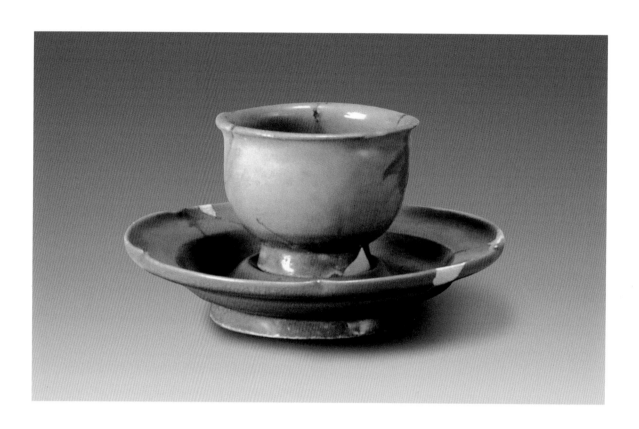

青釉瓷盏托

五代后周

瓷质

盏：口径 8.4 厘米，足径 4.8 厘米，盏高 6 厘米

托：口径 15 厘米，足径 8.5 厘米，高 3 厘米

Celadon-glazed Cup and Saucer

Late Zhou Dynasty of the Five Dynasties

Porcelain

Cup: Mouth Diameter 8.4 cm/ Foot Diameter 4.8 cm/ Height 6 cm

Saucer: Mouth Diameter 15 cm/ Foot Diameter 8.5 cm/ Height 3 cm

托形似盘，浅斜壁，托心凹下，以置杯足，圈
足外撇。盏侈口，圆唇，腹底下部渐收，圈足
外撇。

陕西省咸阳市彬县文化馆藏

The plate-shaped saucer was designed with
shallow oblique wall, a concaved bottom for
holding the cup, and a flared circular foot. With
a slightly flared mouth and a ring foot, the cup
has a round rim and an abdomen narrowing
down gradually.
Preserved in the Cultural Centre of Bin County,
Xianyang, Shaanxi Province

索 引

（馆藏地按拼音字母排序）

中国国家博物馆

中华医学会 / 上海中医药大学医史博物馆

Index

参考文献

[1] 李经纬 . 中国古代医史图录 [M]. 北京：人民卫生出版社，1992.

[2] 傅维康，李经纬，林昭庚 . 中国医学通史：文物图谱卷 [M]. 北京：人民卫生出版社，2000.

[3] 和中浚，吴鸿洲 . 中华医学文物图集 [M]. 成都：四川人民出版社，2001.

[4] 上海中医药博物馆 . 上海中医药博物馆馆藏珍品 [M]. 上海：上海科学技术出版社，2013.

[5] 西藏自治区博物馆 . 西藏博物馆 [M]. 北京：五洲传播出版社，2005.

[6] 崔乐泉 . 中国古代体育文物图录：中英文本 [M]. 北京：中华书局，2000.

[7] 张金明，陆雪春 . 中国古铜镜鉴赏图录 [M]. 北京：中国民族摄影艺术出版社，2002.

[8] 文物精华编辑委员会 . 文物精华 [M]. 北京：文物出版社，1964.

[9] 谭维四 . 湖北出土文物精华 [M]. 武汉：湖北教育出版社，2001.

[10] 常州市博物馆 . 常州文物精华 [M]. 北京：文物出版社，1998.

[11] 镇江博物馆 . 镇江文物精华 [M]. 合肥：黄山书社，1997.

[12] 贵州省文化厅，贵州省博物馆 . 贵州文物精华 [M]. 贵阳：贵州人民出版社，2005.

[13] 徐良玉 . 扬州馆藏文物精华 [M]. 南京：江苏古籍出版社，2001.

[14] 昭陵博物馆，陕西历史博物馆 . 昭陵文物精华 [M]. 西安：陕西人民美术出版社，1991.

[15] 南通博物苑 . 南通博物苑文物精华 [M]. 北京：文物出版社，2005.

[16] 邯郸市文物研究所 . 邯郸文物精华 [M]. 北京：文物出版社，2005.

[17] 张秀生，刘友恒，聂连顺，等 . 中国河北正定文物精华 [M]. 北京：文化艺术出版社，1998.

[18] 陕西省咸阳市文物局 . 咸阳文物精华 [M]. 北京：文物出版社，2002.

[19] 安阳市文物管理局 . 安阳文物精华 [M]. 北京：文物出版社，2004.

[20] 深圳市博物馆 . 深圳市博物馆文物精华 [M]. 北京：文物出版社，1998.

[21]《中国文物精华》编辑委员会 . 中国文物精华（1993）[M]. 北京：文物出版社，1993.

[22] 夏路，刘永生．山西省博物馆馆藏文物精华 [M]．太原：山西人民出版社，1999．

[23] 文物精华编辑委员会．文物精华 [M]．文物出版社，1957．

[24] 山西博物院，湖北省博物馆．荆楚长歌：九连墩楚墓出土文物精华 [M]．太原：山西人民出版社，2011．

[25] 刘广堂，石金鸣，宋建忠．晋国雄风：山西出土两周文物精华 [M]．沈阳：万卷出版公司，2009．

[26] 沈君山，王国平，单迎红．滦平博物馆馆藏文物精华 [M]．北京：中国文联出版社，2012．

[27] 张家口市博物馆．张家口市博物馆馆藏文物精华 [M]．北京：科学出版社，2011．

[28] 浙江省文物考古研究所．浙江考古精华 [M]．北京：文物出版社，1999．

[29] 故宫博物院．故宫雕刻珍萃 [M]．北京：紫禁城出版社，2004．

[30] 故宫博物院紫禁城出版社．故宫博物院藏宝录 [M]．上海：上海文艺出版社，1986．

[31] 首都博物馆．大元三都 [M]．北京：科学出版社，2016．

[32] 新疆维吾尔自治区博物馆．新疆出土文物 [M]．北京：文物出版社，1975．

[33] 王兴伊，段逸山．新疆出土涉医文书辑校 [M]．上海：上海科学技术出版社，2016．

[34] 刘学春．刍议医药卫生文物的概念与分类标准 [J]．中华中医药杂志，2016，31（11）:4406-4409．

[35] 上海古籍出版社．中国艺海 [M]．上海：上海古籍出版社，1994．

[36] 紫都，岳鑫．一生必知的 200 件国宝 [M]．呼和浩特：远方出版社，2005．

[37] 谭维四．湖北出土文物精华 [M]．武汉：湖北教育出版社，2001．

[38] 张建青．青海彩陶收藏与鉴赏 [M]．北京：中国文史出版社，2007．

[39] 银景琦．仡佬族文物 [M]．南宁：广西人民出版社，2014．

[40] 廖果，梁峻，李经纬．东西方医学的反思与前瞻 [M]．北京：中医古籍出版社，2002．

[41] 梁峻，张志斌，廖果，等．中华医药文明史集论 [M]．北京：中医古籍出版社，2003．

[42] 郑蓉，庄乾竹，刘聪，等．中国医药文化遗产考论 [M]．北京：中医古籍出版社，2005．